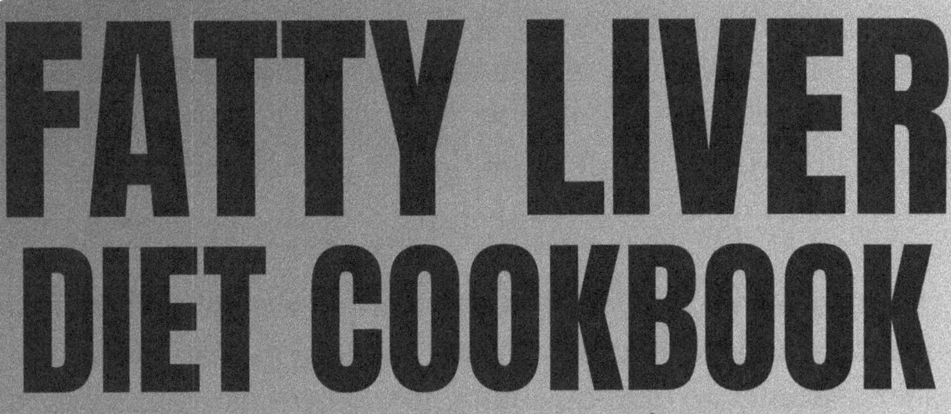

FATTY LIVER
DIET COOKBOOK
For Beginners and Seniors

Delicious and Easy-to-Cook Low-Fat Recipes To
Help You Detoxify and Reverse Fatty Liver

+

28-Day
MEAL PLAN

**ANTI-INFLAMMATORY EATING
COOKBOOK**

**2024
EDITION**

JUANITA SCOTT

Copyright © 2023 Juanita Scott

● ● ●

Disclaimer

The information provided in this book is for general informational purposes only. It is not intended to be a substitute for professional medical advice, diagnosis, or treatment. Always seek the advice of your physician or other qualified health provider with any questions you may have regarding a medical condition.

The author and publisher of this book have made every effort to ensure that the information in this book is accurate and up-to-date at the time of publication. However, they make no representations or warranties of any kind, express or implied, about the completeness, accuracy, reliability, suitability, or availability of the information contained within. The author and publisher disclaim any responsibility for any adverse effects or consequences resulting from the use of the information presented in this book.

The dietary recommendations and recipes provided in this book are intended as general guidelines and may not be suitable for everyone. Individual nutritional needs vary, and it is advisable to consult with a qualified healthcare professional or registered dietitian before making significant changes to your diet.

This book may contain references to specific products, services, or third-party websites. These references are provided for informational purposes only and do not constitute an endorsement or recommendation.

Juanita Scott
Juanitascott007@gmail.com

About the Author

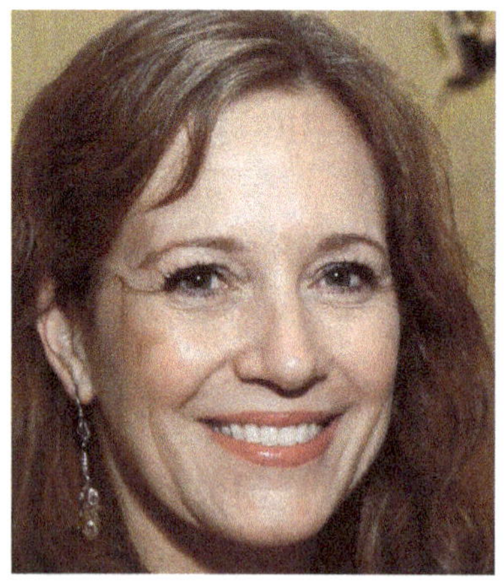

Meet Juanita Scott, a culinary virtuoso, seasoned nutritionist, and dedicated dietitian whose passion for healthy eating and lifestyle has transformed the lives of many. Beyond the artistry of the kitchen, Juanita brings a wealth of expertise, seamlessly blending her culinary mastery with a deep understanding of nutrition to create a holistic approach to well-being.

With years of experience as a chef, Juanita has honed her skills in crafting not only delectable meals but also dishes that prioritize health without compromising on flavor. Her culinary creations are a testament to the belief that nutritious food can be both a source of nourishment and a celebration of taste.

As an accomplished nutritionist and dietitian, Juanita goes beyond the realm of recipes, weaving together the intricate dance of nutrients and their impact on overall health. Her commitment to promoting wellness extends beyond the pages of cookbooks, resonating in every piece of advice she shares with her audience.

Married and blessed with a beautiful family, Juanita understands the importance of fostering a lifestyle that caters to the needs of both adults and children. Her family-friendly approach to healthy living is reflected not only in her recipes but also in the way she encourages households to embrace wellness as a shared journey.

Juanita's unique perspective on the symbiosis of culinary art and nutritional science makes her a sought-after authority in the realm of healthy living. Her work has inspired countless individuals to reevaluate their relationship with food, transforming meals into moments of nourishment, joy, and familial connection.

When she's not in the kitchen or counseling clients, Juanita revels in the simple pleasures of family life. Her dedication to her own family's health echoes in the heartfelt advice and delicious recipes she shares with readers.

Join Juanita Scott on a journey to a revitalized, healthier you. Through her books, consultations, and culinary creations, she invites you to savor the richness of life and health, one mindful bite at a time.

Table Of Contents

Introduction

Amidst the peaceful stretches of her golden years, my dear friend Helen encountered an unanticipated foe: non-alcoholic fatty liver disease (NAFLD). It was a diagnosis that cast doubt on her previously tranquil life. A regular examination had revealed something she wasn't ready to face.

The diagnosis came to her as she sat in the cold, clinical light of the physician's office: "Helen, you have non-alcoholic fatty liver disease. It's a condition that needs to be managed, but we can control it with the correct lifestyle adjustments."

Helen asked for my assistance because she was confused and afraid, and we set out to discover the truth about this silent invader that had taken up residence in her liver. She quickly discovered that NAFLD required close observation since it frequently showed no symptoms at first. She had no idea that years of seemingly innocuous eating patterns and a sedentary lifestyle had prepared the ground for this unwanted visitor.

But Helen and I saw a glimmer of hope in the diagnosis: a diet high in fatty liver that might be able to turn the tide. She went headfirst into the world of liver-friendly nutrition, fearless and determined to take back control of her health. The days of careless excess were over, and she welcomed a brand-new culinary journey.

Equipped with her newfound knowledge, Helen made her way through the grocery store aisles and came across a color and flavor palette that would eventually turn out to be her ally. Her regular meals were now composed of crisp vegetables, colorful fruits, lean proteins, and whole grains.

Once a place of convenience, the kitchen became a haven of healing for her. Helen and I played around with meals that were a celebration of flavor as much as they were nutritious. Every meal was a deliberate decision, a step toward healing her liver and, consequently, her entire health.

Weeks became months, and Helen's lifestyle modifications, albeit little at first, had a significant impact. The good transformation within was reflected in the follow-up sessions with her healthcare practitioner, which was none other than me. Tests for liver function revealed improvements, and the threat posed by NAFLD started to fade.

Through the process, Helen found a deep shift in perspective in addition to a diet. The diet for fatty liver was a route to vitality rather than a restrictive schedule. It involved enthusiastically saying "yes" to a healthier, more active life rather than merely saying "no" to particular meals.

My ten-year journey culminated in this book, which is a monument to the strength of wise decisions and the human spirit's resiliency. I hope that this culinary journey we are on together will serve as an inspiration to everyone who wants to feed their livers and enjoy life to the fullest.

Understanding Fatty Liver Disease

There are chapters in the complex story of our health that frequently come as a surprise. One such surprising discovery for many is the diagnosis of alcohol-related fatty liver disease (ALD) or non-alcoholic fatty liver disease (NAFLD). This chapter provides an overview of the condition's complexities as well as the empowering process of comprehending and controlling it with a diet that promotes fatty liver.

Once overshadowed by its alcoholic cousin, fatty liver disease has gained widespread attention in the last few years. It is a disorder where too much fat builds up in the liver as a result of sedentary lifestyle choices and poor nutritional choices in addition to alcohol usage.

It's critical to understand the nuances of fatty liver disease as we begin this exploration. Imagine the liver, that tenacious organ that sits beneath our ribs and does a multitude of tasks that are vital to our health. Imagine it now progressively gaining fat, frequently without any outward signs or sound.

Peeling back the layers of causation—from genetics to metabolic variables, insulin resistance to obesity—is necessary to understand fatty liver. Every piece of the jigsaw adds to the total picture of liver health. Seniors in particular are at a turning point in their lives where all of their life's decisions come together.

This chapter explores the basic causes and mechanisms of fatty liver disease. It's an exploration of the maze of medical knowledge, transforming technical jargon into an engaging story that gives readers power over information. It is the compass that directs us toward making wise decisions, and when it comes to fatty liver, it may be a powerful instrument for transformation.

What is Fatty Liver Disease?

An excess of fat in the liver is known as fatty liver. It is prevalent, especially in individuals with diabetes and excess weight. It may not show any symptoms, yet it can result in serious health issues. The disorder can be prevented and improved by making lifestyle modifications.

The primary organ in the body for breaking down food and waste is the liver. There is either very little or no fat in a healthy liver. When you consume excessive amounts of food or alcohol, your body responds by storing some of the excess energy as fat. The cells in the liver then store this fat.

You have fatty liver when fat accounts for more than 5–10% of your liver's total weight. The prevalence of fatty liver is rising with the use of additional carbohydrates and fats. In Australia, fatty liver disease affects about one in three adult citizens.

Symptoms Of Fatty Liver Disease?

Most of the time, fatty liver disease is asymptomatic. Individuals exhibiting symptoms could:
- Feel worn out or generally sick
- Experience abdominal ache in the upper right section.
- Reduce in weight

The following are indicators that you might have more severe fatty liver disease:
- Jaundice (yellow eyes and skin)
- bruising
- dark urination
- bloated stomach
- vomiting blood
- Black stools (poos)
- Skin irritation

If you experience any of these signs, consult your physician.

What Causes Fatty Liver Disease?

Usually, several variables working together over an extended period result in fatty liver.

The following are the main reasons for fatty liver:
- Being overweight or obese, particularly in the abdomen (tummy)
- Having insulin resistance or type 2 diabetes
- Having elevated triglycerides or cholesterol in the blood
- Overindulging in alcohol consumption

Less frequently occurring reasons include:
- Hypothyroidism
- Some medications
- Having PCOS (polycystic ovarian syndrome)
- Late-stage pregnancy difficulties can also induce fatty liver in certain individuals.

Types of Fatty Liver Diseases

Fat-related liver disease comes in two primary forms:

1. **Nonalcoholic fatty liver disease (NAFLD)**

In the United States, one in three persons has this form of disease. Although the specific reason is unknown, obesity and diabetes will raise your chance of contracting it. You don't get it from drinking alcohol, in contrast to the other main variety. NAFLD comes in two forms:

Simple fatty liver: Refers to the presence of fat in the liver without any associated liver cell injury or inflammation. Usually, it doesn't worsen or result in liver issues. The majority of NAFLD patients have basic fatty livers.

Nonalcoholic steatohepatitis (NASH): Compared to simple fatty liver, this condition is far more dangerous. NASH indicates that your liver is inflamed. NASH-related inflammation and liver cell destruction can lead to major issues such as liver cancer and the scarring conditions of cirrhosis and fibrosis. Liver failure brought on by these issues may necessitate a liver transplant. NASH affects about 20% of patients with NAFLD.

2. **Alcohol-related fatty liver disease (ALD)**

This type, which affects roughly 5% of Americans, is less frequent and is brought on by alcohol consumption. Because of this, things normally get better when you cut back on alcohol. If you continue to drink, ALD may result in major issues. Among them are:

Enlarged liver. You might have pain or discomfort on the upper right side of your abdomen, though symptoms aren't usually present.

Alcoholic hepatitis. This is an enlargement of the liver that can result in fever, vomiting, nausea, abdominal pain, and jaundice (yellow eyes and skin).

Alcoholic Cirrhosis. This is a hepatic accumulation of scar tissue. Along with the same symptoms as alcoholic hepatitis, it can also cause:

- Large-scale fluid accumulation in your abdomen, which your

- doctor will refer to as ascites.
- Elevated hepatic blood pressure
- Bleeding internally
- Perplexity and behavioral shifts
- Enlarged spleen, a little immune system organ located inside the rib cage
- A deadly liver failure can occur.
- Fatty liver disease associated with alcohol usually occurs first. After that, it may worsen and develop into alcoholic hepatitis. It could develop into alcoholic cirrhosis over time.

Discuss your drinking habits with your physician if you drink heavily. They can help you control your drinking to preserve your health, and it's discreet.

Risk Factors for Fatty Liver Disease

Alcohol overindulgence is the root cause of ALD. You may be even more likely to get it if you drink a lot and;
- Are overweight
- Are undernourished
- Having persistent viral hepatitis, particularly hepatitis C
- Possess masculine anatomy or are African American or Hispanic guy
- Because of the way women digest alcohol, they are either female or have female anatomy.
- Age-related: the likelihood increases with age

It is unknown why some NAFLD patients develop simple fatty liver while others develop nonalcoholic steatosis (NASH). Genes could be the cause. NASH or NAFLD is more probable if:
- You are overweight or obese.
- Insulin resistance is the state in which your body does not respond to insulin as it should, or if you have type 2 diabetes.
- You either have low amounts of "good" (HDL) cholesterol or high levels of triglycerides or "bad" (LDL) cholesterol.
- You're more mature.

- The syndrome of polycystic ovary
- That's sleep apnea.
- Your doctor will refer to your underactive thyroid as hypothyroidism.
- Your pituitary gland is underactive; this condition is known as hypopituitarism.
- You've had rapid weight loss. You're malnourished.
- You've come into contact with some chemicals and toxins.
- Are you Asian or Hispanic?
- Metabolic syndrome is what you have. Type 2 diabetes and heart disease are more likely to develop in people with this combination of diseases. If you have metabolic syndrome, you could have any one of these three ailments:
- Large waist measurement
- high LDL cholesterol or triglycerides
- Low HDL (good) cholesterol levels
- Elevated blood pressure
- Elevated blood sugar

Additionally, there are a few less frequent causes of NAFLD and NASH. Among them are:
- Diseases that alter how fat is used or stored by the body
- Other infections, such as hepatitis C
- Quick decrease in weight
- Utilizing specific medications, such synthetic estrogen, glucocorticoids, methotrexate (Rheumatrex, Trexall), tamoxifen (Nolvadex, Soltamox), and others
- Gallbladder removal. There is a higher chance of NAFLD in certain patients who undergo surgery to remove their gallbladder.

Handling Adipose Liver Disease

While some are under clinical studies, there are currently no authorized medicines for NAFLD.

Losing weight is usually the initial course of treatment: It aids in the reduction of liver scarring, inflammation, and fat. The amount of fat in your liver can be reduced by losing as little as 3% to 5% of your body weight. If you are overweight, surgery is another possibility for you.

You will also have to give up alcohol: It is the only approach to prevent the worsening of liver damage. Even some of the liver damage that has already occurred might be repairable. Discuss with your physician how you might obtain assistance. To safely stop drinking and manage the symptoms of withdrawal, you might require a detox program under medical supervision.

In the event that you develop NASH-related problems such as liver failure or cirrhosis, you might require a liver transplant. People with NASH who receive a liver transplant typically recover greatly.

Alternative Therapies for Fatty Liver Disease

Vitamin E: Research has indicated that vitamin E may help liver health by decreasing inflammation; however, the effects differed according to the patient's age, weight, and dosage. Furthermore, several researches suggested that those with FLD and other medical disorders may be at risk from excessive vitamin E dosages.

Coffee: It has long been believed that caffeine helps the liver and can reduce the amount of scarring caused by a *Variety of liver illnesses:* How coffee protects the liver is unknown. Coffee is thought to stimulate liver-cleansing enzymes. Coffee also contains chemicals that reduce inflammation.

Olive oil: Olive oil is a healthy fat that decreases inflammation, enhances your body's ability to process fats and carbohydrates after a meal, and lessens the quantity of fat deposited in your liver.

Since research on all of these products is ongoing, consult a physician or nutritionist before deciding to take extra vitamin E or olive oil or drink more coffee every day.

Reversing Fatty Liver Disease

You can reverse fatty liver disease by quitting alcohol and losing weight. One of the few organs in the body that has the ability to regenerate damaged tissue instead of leaving scars behind is the liver. However, the reversal is only effective if you stop consuming alcohol and unhealthy diets.

Self-Care for Fatty Liver Disease
These lifestyle changes can help:

Get more exercise: Make an effort to exercise for at least half an hour most days of the week. You may discover that exercising beyond this helps if you're attempting to lose weight. However, if you don't currently exercise frequently, start out carefully and ask for your doctor's approval beforehand.

Treat your liver with kindness: Avoid actions that will increase its workload. Give up booze. Adhere to the directions on prescription and over-the-counter medications. Consult your physician before using any natural therapies. Because a product is natural does not mean is safe for you.

Reduce your cholesterol: Take your meds on time, exercise, and eat a plant-based diet. This will raise and maintain the appropriate levels of triglycerides and cholesterol.

Control your blood sugar: Monitor your blood sugar levels and follow your doctor's prescriptions for medication.

A buildup of fat in the liver is known as fatty liver disease. Alcohol consumption is one cause of this illness. The other, more prevalent kind has no known cause, although conditions like diabetes and obesity can raise your chance of developing it. Fortunately, lifestyle modifications including improving your diet, exercising, and cutting back on alcohol can lessen or even repair liver damage.

polyphenolic content of spinach and other leafy greens.

Soy and Beans to Lower the Risk of NAFLD
Soy and beans have both demonstrated potential in lowering the risk of NAFLD. Legumes, including lentils, chickpeas, soybeans, and peas, are high in nutrients and also include resistant starches that support gut health, according to a scholarly review of diet and liver disease.

Legumes can even help persons who are obese reduce their lipids and blood sugar. Furthermore, a 2019 study discovered that diets high in legumes particularly reduced the risk of NAFLD. Though the data is conflicting, a few studies have also suggested that eating soy—whether it be in the form of fermented soy soup or as a substitute for meat or fish—may help preserve the liver.

This is most likely due to soy's high β-conglycinin protein concentration, which is known to help decrease triglyceride levels and may even defend against the formation of visceral fat. Tofu is also a low-fat item that is a great source of protein, which makes it a great option if you're attempting to cut back on your fat intake.

Fish, Helps Reduce Fat and Inflammatory Levels
Omega-3 fatty acids are abundant in fatty fish, including trout, sardines, salmon, and tuna.

According to research, taking an omega-3 supplement may help people with NAFLD by lowering triglyceride levels, increasing beneficial HDL cholesterol, and decreasing liver fat.

Fiber-Rich Whole Grains
Oatmeal and other whole-grain, high-fiber diets are linked to a lower risk of disorders related to non-alcoholic fatty liver disease (NAFLD).

According to studies, people with NAFLD can benefit from a healthy diet high in high-fiber foods like oats, which can also lower triglyceride levels.

Nuts to Help as an Anti-inflammatory

Reduced oxidative stress, insulin resistance, inflammation, and the prevalence of NAFLD are linked to a diet high in nuts.

Increased nut consumption was found to be significantly connected with a lowered risk of nonalcoholic fatty liver disease (NAFLD) in a large Chinese study. Additionally, eating walnuts has been linked to improved liver function tests in individuals with fatty liver disease.

Using Turmeric to Lower Liver Damage Indicators
The active component of turmeric, curcumin, may lessen liver damage markers in NAFLD patients when taken in high amounts.

Turmeric has been shown in studies to lower serum levels of two enzymes that are excessively elevated in patients with fatty liver disease: aspartate aminotransferase (AST) and alanine aminotransferase (ALT). These studies focus on the supplementation of turmeric.

Antioxidants From Sunflower Seeds
Particularly rich in vitamin E, sunflower nuts are a popular antioxidant supplement for NAFLD patients.

Although the majority of studies on NAFLD and vitamin E concentrate on supplements, a 100-gram portion of sunflower seeds contains around 20 mg of vitamin E, which is more than 100% of the Daily Recommended Value. Sunflower seeds are a great place to start if you want to organically increase your vitamin E intake.

Eat More Unsaturated Fat
For people with non-alcoholic fatty liver disease (NAFLD), replacing sources of saturated fat (such as butter, fatty meat cuts, sausages, and cured meats) with unsaturated fat (such as avocados, olive oil, nut butter, and fatty fish) may be beneficial.

This is one of the reasons the Mediterranean diet, which emphasizes minimally processed whole foods high in fruits, vegetables, and legumes and low in unsaturated fat, is sometimes suggested for people with non-alcoholic fatty liver disease (NAFLD). The diet also helps lower total cholesterol levels.

Garlic for General Health Improvement

In addition to giving food flavor, a few small experimental studies suggest that supplementing with garlic powder may help reduce body weight and fat in individuals with fatty liver disease.

A recent 2020 study found that taking 800 mg of garlic powder daily for 15 weeks decreased liver fat and increased enzyme levels in individuals with NAFLD. In terms of whole food intake, a 2019 study discovered that regular raw garlic consumption in Chinese men was inversely correlated with non-alcoholic fatty liver disease (NAFLD) (but not in women).

Foods To Limit Or Avoid

If you have fatty liver disease, your doctor may advise you to avoid specific foods, or to take them in moderation. These foods, in general, contribute to weight gain and can raise blood sugar levels.

When possible, avoid:
- Alcohol. Alcohol is a major contributor to fatty liver disease and other liver illnesses.
- Sugar has been added. Sugary foods such as candies, cookies, sodas, and fruit juices should be avoided. High blood sugar levels increase the amount of fat that accumulates in the liver.
- Foods that have been fried. These include a lot of fat and calories.
- Excessive salt consumption. Excessive salt consumption can raise the risk of NAFLD. It is advised to reduce sodium intake to less than 2,300 mg per day. High blood pressure patients should limit their salt consumption to no more than 1,500 mg per day.
- White bread, rice, and spaghetti are all options. Because of the lack of fiber in white flour, things cooked with it can spike your blood sugar more than whole grains.
- Meat that is red. Saturated fat is abundant in beef and pork. Highly processed meats in general (sausage, pepperoni, bacon, and so on) should also be avoided because they are rich in sodium and saturated fat.

If you have NAFLD or are at risk of having it, certain lifestyle and nutritional modifications can help improve the health of your liver and lower your chance of developing it.

The greatest strategy to improve liver function, minimize disease risk, and support healthy weight reduction is to eat a well-balanced, nutritional diet high in fiber, lean or plant-based protein, and healthy fats.

If you have NAFLD or are concerned that you might have it, consult with a trusted healthcare provider to develop a treatment plan that includes dietary adjustments as well as lifestyle improvements such as increasing physical activity, improving sleep, and reducing stress.

Breakfast Boosters

1. Chia seeds pudding

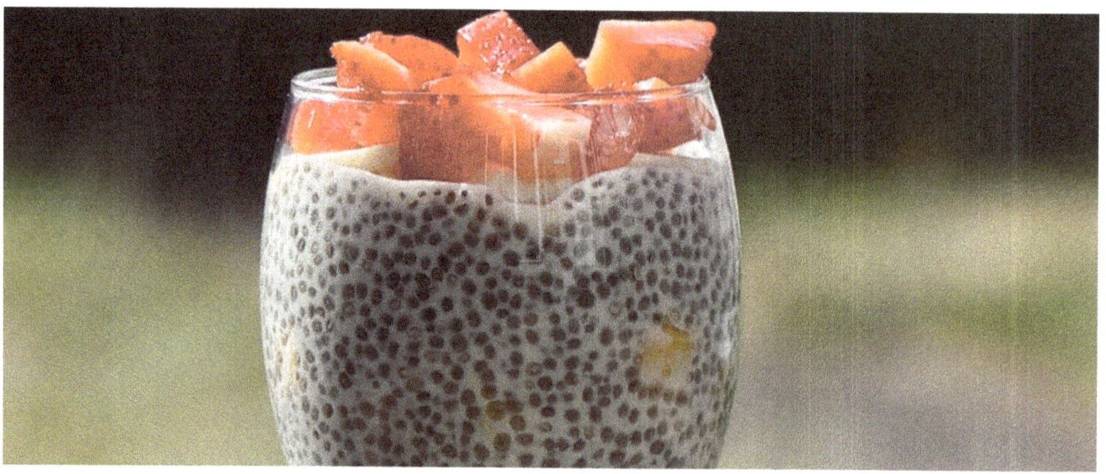

Ingredients:

- Four tablespoons of chia seeds
- One cup almond milk or your preferred milk
- Two tsp honey, or alternative sweetener, if desired
- Strawberries or additional fruits as a garnish

Nutritional Value

- Calories: 155 kcal
- Carbohydrate: 16g
- Fats: 9g
- Protein: 5g

Instructions:

- Combine items in a container and stir thoroughly.
- Allow to sit for two to three minutes, then thoroughly mix once more until no clumps are visible.
- Place the jar in the refrigerator for at least two hours or overnight, covered.
- When it's time to eat, garnish with your preferred fruit and consume it chilled!

Prep Time: 5mins   **Serves:** 2

Freeze Time: 2hrs

Total Time: 2hr 5mins

2. Fruit salad

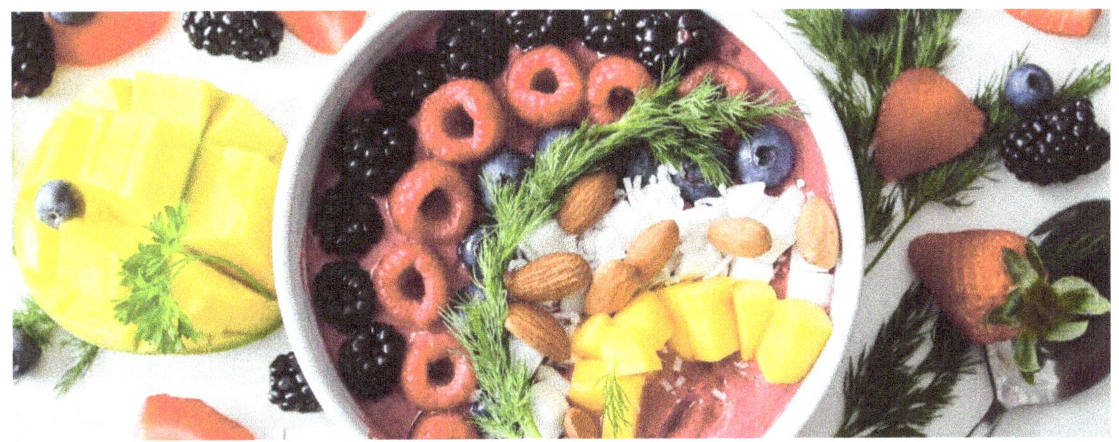

Ingredients:

For the Dressing
- ¼ cup honey
- ¼ cup of recently extracted orange juice
- one lemon's zest

For the Salad
- One pound of quartered and hulled strawberries
- Six ounces of blueberries
- Six ounces of raspberries
- 3 sliced and peeled kiwis
- One orange, peeled and sliced into half wedges
- Two apples, cut and peeled
- One mango, cut and peeled
- 2 c. grapes

Nutritional Value (10 cups)

- Calories: 142 kcal
- Carbohydrate: 32g
- Fats: 1g
- Protein: 2g

Instructions:

1. In a small bowl, make sure to combine the orange juice, honey and the lemon zest.
2. Place the fruit in a big bowl, then add the dressing and carefully stir to mix.
3. Chill until ready to serve.

Prep Time: 15mins **Serves: 8-10**

Cooking Time: 0 mins

Total Time: 20ins

3. Guacamole Toast

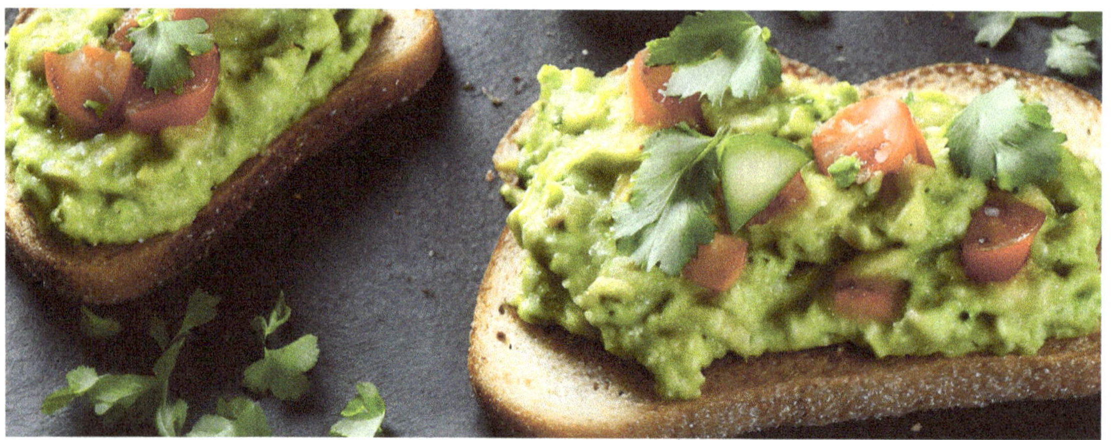

Ingredients:

- One medium avocado
- ½ lemon or lime that has been juiced
- Salt and pepper to taste
- One teaspoon of sesame seeds
- Two slices Food for Life Flourless Sprouted Grain Bread

Nutritional Value

- Calories: 168 kcal
- Carbohydrate: 20g
- Fats: 9g
- Protein: 4g

Instructions:

1. Mash the avocado and season with salt, pepper, and lemon or lime juice.
2. Cover the bread with the avocado mixture.
3. As desired, scatter sesame seeds.

Prep Time: 5mins   **Serves:** 2

Cooking Time: 0min

Total Time: 10mins

4. Homemade Oatmeal

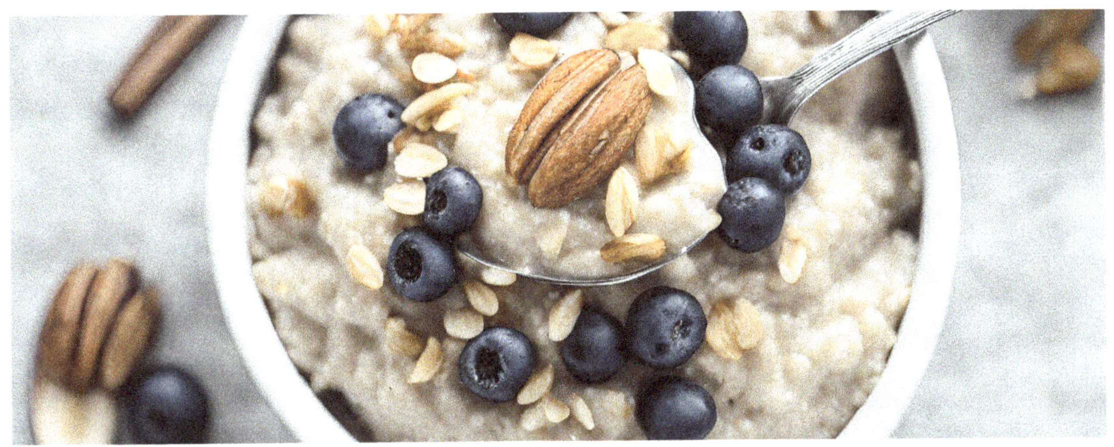

Ingredients:

- one cup of water
- half a cup of rolled oats
- One tablespoon of chia seeds
- Two tablespoons of hemp seeds
- Half a teaspoon of cinnamon
- ¾ cup almond milk
- 1 tsp coconut sugar

Nutritional Value

- Calories: ~340.5kcal
- Carbohydrate: ~40.75g
- Fats: ~15.3g
- Protein: ~14.75g

Instructions:

1. Measure and pour in one cup of water and heat to a boil in a pot.
2. Add the hemp seeds, chia, and oats to the boiling water. Cook, stirring periodically, for 3 minutes.
3. Transfer to a bowl and garnish with coconut sugar, cinnamon, and almond milk.

Prep Time: 2mins   **Serves: 1**
Cooking Time: 3mins
Total Time: 5mins

5. Greek Yogurt and Berries

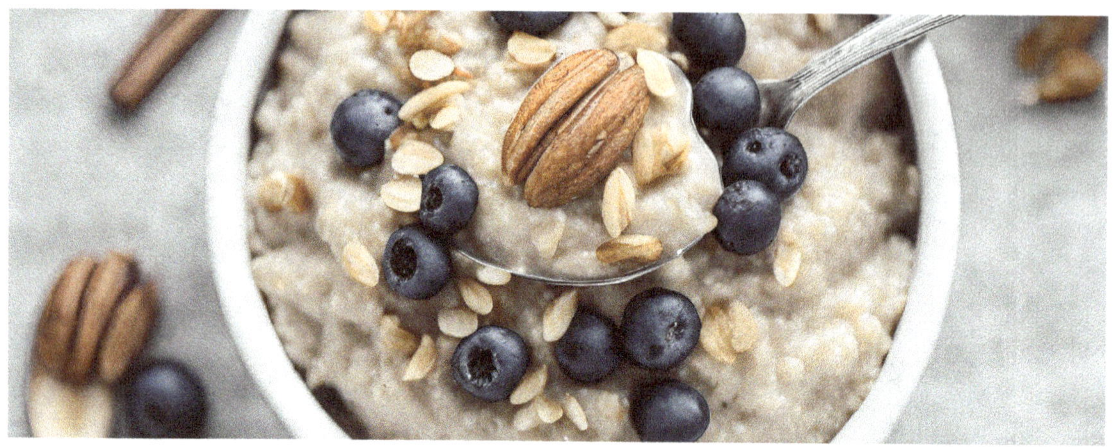

Ingredients:

- ¾ cup of Greek yogurt
- Half cup of blueberries
- one cup of strawberries, chopped
- One tablespoon of honey

Nutritional Value

- Calories: 240 kcal
- Carbohydrate: 44g
- Fats: 1g
- Protein: 16g

Instructions:

1. In a bowl, put ¾ cup of yogurt.
2. After washing and slicing the berries, arrange them over the yogurt.
3. Overtop, drizzle some honey. Savor it as a delicious breakfast

Prep Time: 5 mins   **Serves: 1**

Cooking Time: 0 mins

Total Time: 5mins

6. Mediterranean Quinoa Salad

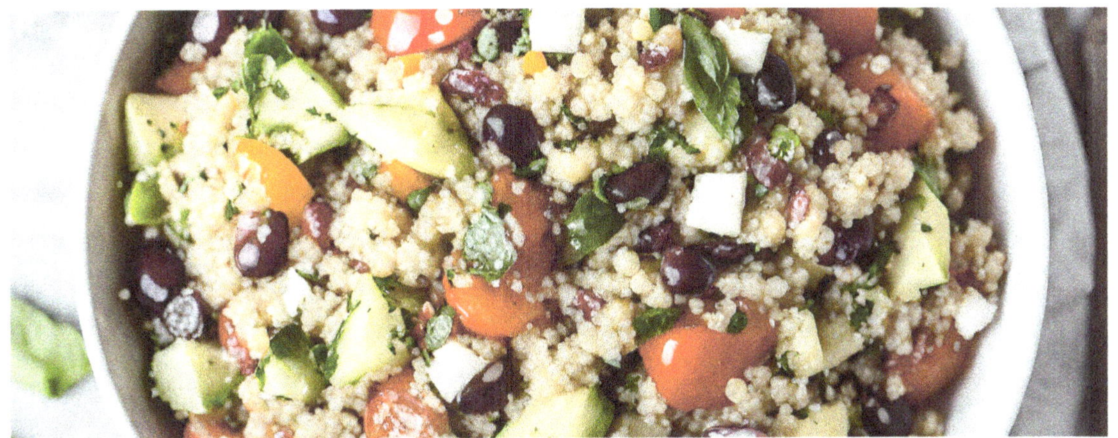

Ingredients:

- Four cups of arugula
- One cup of cooked quinoa
- One cup of cooked, chopped beets (ideally organic)
- One fifteen-oz can of rinsed and drained chickpeas

For The Dressing

- One lemon's juice
- 2 tablespoons tahini
- One tablespoon of mustard, coarsely chopped
- One grated clove of garlic
- One tablespoon of water, if necessary
- To taste, add salt and pepper.

Nutritional Value

- Calories: 475 kcal
- Carbohydrate: 71g
- Fats: 14g
- Protein: 19g

Instructions:

- All salad ingredients should be mixed together in a big bowl.
- Mix the ingredients for the vinaigrette using a whisk. Add the salad and toss to mix everything well.
- Serve right away or refrigerate for 30 minutes (optional).

Prep Time: 5 mins   **Serves:** 2

Cooking Time: 15 mins

Total Time: 20 mins

7. Fresh Vegetable Salad

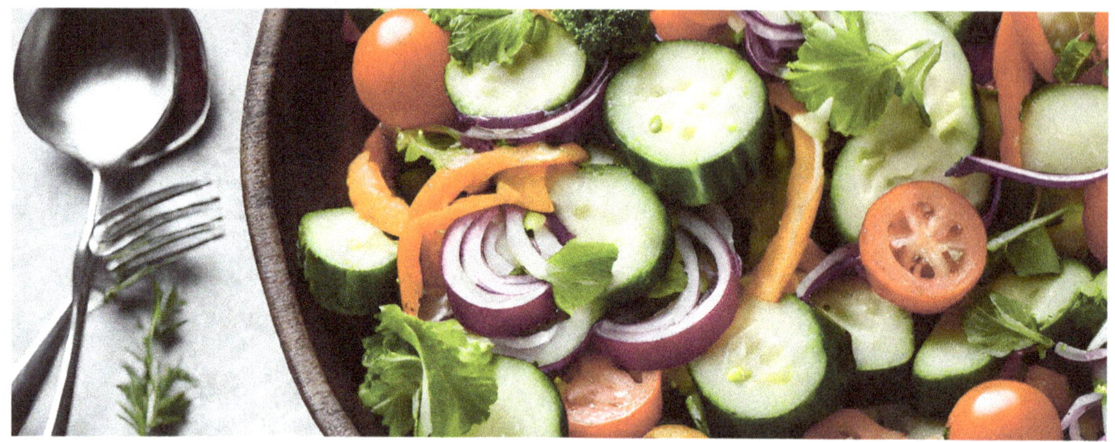

Ingredients:

- 3-4 small field cucumbers or ⅓ English cucumber, chopped
- 1 cup cherry tomatoes.
- 1 red bell pepper, split in half,
- 9 cored and diced radishes, chopped
- 2-3 celery stalks, diced
- ⅓ medium onion, thinly sliced
- 2-3 garlic cloves, minced
- 1 large handful fresh parsley, chopped
- 1 generous handful fresh dill
- 2 tablespoons balsamic vinegar
- 3 tablespoons olive oil
- salt to taste

Instructions:

- Place all of the vegetables and herbs in a salad bowl.
- Combine the balsamic vinegar and olive oil in a small bowl and drizzle over the vegetables.
- Toss with salt and pepper to taste. Refrigerate for 30 minutes to enable the flavors to meld.

Prep Time: 5 mins   **Serves: 4-5**

Cooking Time: 15 mins

Total Time: 20 mins

Nutritional Value

- Calories: 162 kcal
- Carbohydrate: 16g
- Fats: 11g   • Protein: 3g

8. Skinny Omelet

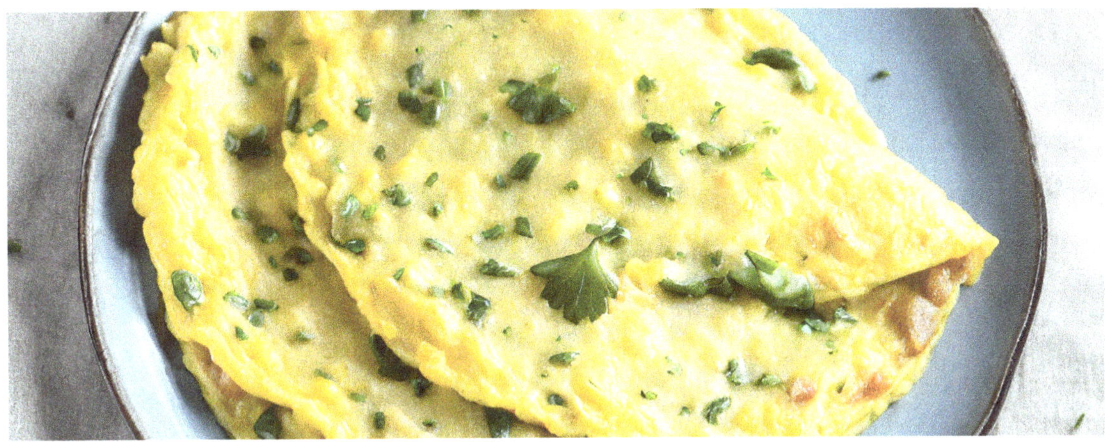

Ingredients:

- 2 beaten big eggs
- a little pinch of fine grain sea salt
- a few tablespoons minced chives or herbs
- a smear of pesto
- a smear of goat cheese or feta
- a smattering of mixed salad greens

Prep Time: 5 mins   **Serves: 1**

Cooking Time: 2mins

Total Time: 7 mins

Nutritional Value

- Calories: 349 kcal
- Carbohydrate: 5g
- Fats: 25g
- Protein: 23g

Instructions:

- Pour the egg mixture into your largest nonstick skillet over medium heat (this is one of the few times I use nonstick) and give it a nice swirl so that it spreads out thinly throughout the entire pan.
- You can also use a crepe pan or crepe maker, which works equally well.
- Sprinkle the eggs with salt and some of the chives and leave aside for 15 seconds to one minute, depending on the heat of your pan. Slide the omelet out of the pan (flat) onto a clean countertop, big cutting

- board, or Silpat-lined cookie sheet with a spatula. Do it with assurance (or practice).
- Spread the pesto across the surface of the omelet (if it's thick, thin it with water to make it easier to spread), then top with the cheese and salad greens.
- Roll the omelet away from you, beginning with one end. Make a deep diagonal cut in half. Season with salt to taste and serve topped with chopped chives and/or other herbs. Serve right away.

9. Healthy Egg Muffins

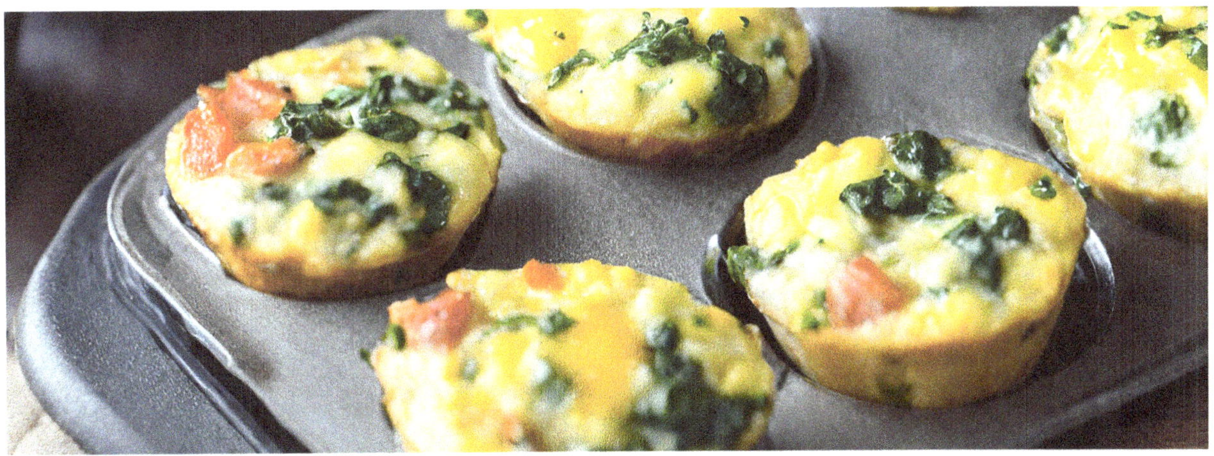

Ingredients:

- 1 tablespoon extra virgin olive oil
- 1 cup red pepper, chopped
- 1 cup green pepper, chopped
- 1 cup yellow onion, chopped
- 2 cups coarsely chopped packed baby spinach
- 1 cup chopped mushrooms
- 2 minced garlic cloves
- Season with salt to taste
- four huge eggs
- 4 egg whites, big
- Optional hot sauce for sprinkling on top!

Prep Time: 10 mins   **Serves: 12**

Cooking Time: 15 mins

Total Time: 25 mins

Instructions:

- Preheat the oven to 350°F and coat a normal nonstick 12-slot muffin pan with cooking spray. Place aside.
- In a large skillet with the heat set to medium, melt the butter.
- When the oil is hot, add the red pepper, green pepper, and onion, and sauté for 5-7 minutes, or until the peppers are cooked, stirring frequently.
- Cook for 2 minutes more after adding the spinach and mushrooms.
- Add the minced garlic in the last 30 seconds.
- Remove from the firc and season with salt.

- In a large 4 cup measuring cup, whisk together the eggs/egg whites until smooth, then add in the cooked vegetables.
- Fill the prepared muffin tin halfway with the egg/veggie mixture, then bake for 15-30 minutes, or until the tops are hard to the touch and the eggs are cooked.
- Allow to cool slightly before serving!

Nutritional Value (1 muffin)

- Calories: 50 kcal
- Carbohydrate: 3g
- Fats: 2g
- Protein: 4g

10. Ricotta Avocado Toast

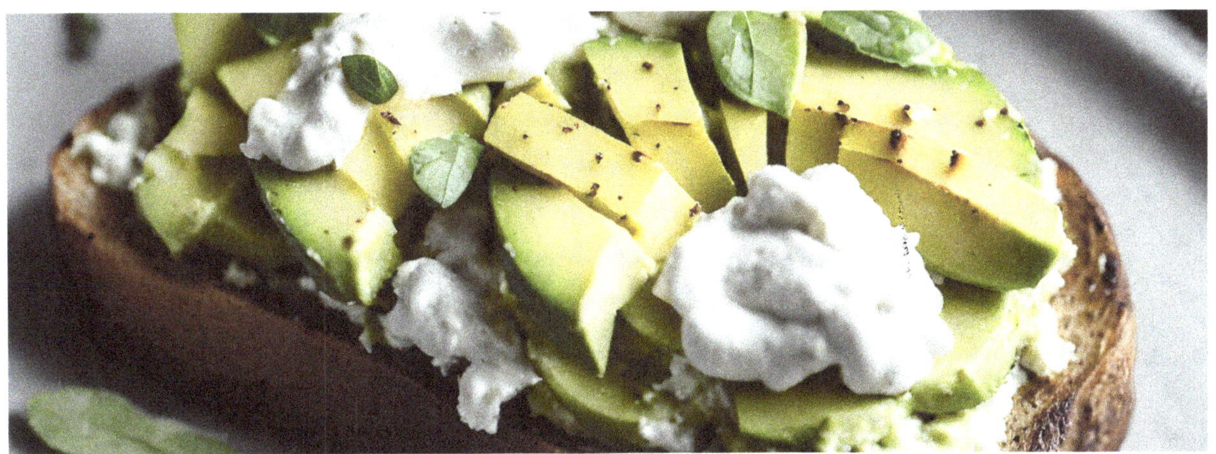

Ingredients:

- 1 slice country or sourdough bread (½ inch thick)
- EVOO (extra virgin olive oil)
- ½ pitted and peeled medium Avocado hash
- ½ lemon, freshly squeezed lemon juice to taste
- 4–5 tbsp. high-quality ricotta
- For garnish, thinly sliced basil leaves
- Lemon zest as a garnish
- Sea salt
- flaky and freshly ground black pepper

Prep Time: 5 mins **Serves:** 1
Cooking Time: 0 mins
Total Time: 5 mins

Instructions:

- Brush bread lightly with extra-virgin olive oil and toast to desired doneness.
- Mash the avocado with a fork to cover the entire surface.
- Squeeze lemon juice over bread and spread dollops of ricotta on top.
- Drizzle with more olive oil and season with basil, lemon zest, sea salt, and pepper.
- Serve.

Nutritional Value

- Calories: 575 kcal
- Carbohydrate: 61g
- Fats: 32g
- Protein: 17g

11. Tofu Scramble

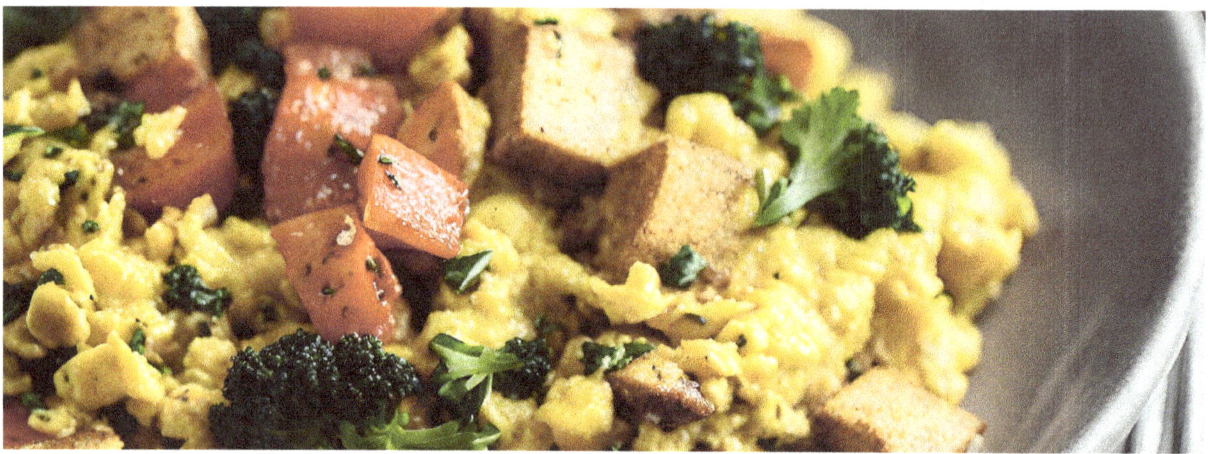

Ingredients:

- 2 teaspoons olive oil, divided—or water if no oil is preferred.
- baby bella mushrooms, 6 oz.
- 1 red pepper, tiny
- three scallions
- 8 oz. firm organic tofu
- 2 tsp. nutritional yeast
- ½ teaspoon turmeric powder
- ¼ tsp garlic powder
- ½ tsp salt
- ½ tsp freshly ground black pepper

Prep Time: 5 mins   **Serves:** 2
Cooking Time: 5 mins
Total Time: 10 mins

Instructions:

- Prepare the vegetables by gently wiping the mushrooms with a damp paper towel and then thinly slicing them. Trim the red pepper and cut it into strips. Scallions should be cut diagonally.
- Tofu should be drained on paper towels before being placed in a bowl. Crumble it into bite-sized pieces using a potato masher or a fork.
- Warm a large skillet over medium heat. Swirl in 1 tablespoon olive oil (you may substitute water here, although you might need a little more), then add mushrooms. Season with salt and pepper. Cook for about 2 minutes, stirring

- occasionally, before adding the red peppers. Before adding the scallions, make to cook for another minute. Set aside the cooked vegetables.
- Swirl in the remaining Tablespoon of olive oil (or water) to the empty side of the pan. Pour in the crumbled tofu, followed by the seasonings. Stir regularly while the tofu cooks and the spices are mixed to turn the tofu from beige to yellow (similar to scrambled eggs). This process should take at least 2 minutes or more.
- Mix the sautéed vegetables with the tofu gently and serve while still warm.

Nutritional Value

- Calories: 275kcal
- Carbohydrate: 13g
- Fats: 20g
- Protein: 16g

12. Vegan Waffles

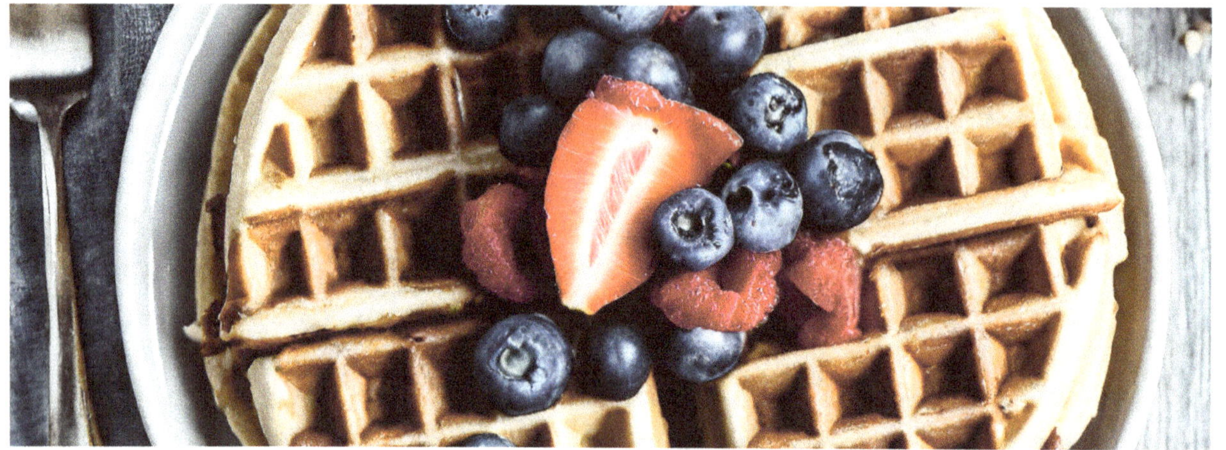

Ingredients:

- 1½ cup unsweetened soy or coconut milk (or any vegan milk)
- 1 tsp apple cider vinegar
- 2 cups (240g) all-purpose flour
- 1 tbsp. baking powder
- ½ teaspoon of sea salt
- 1 tbsp brown sugar (or maple syrup)
- ¼ cup melted coconut oil (or vegan butter)
- ½ teaspoon vanilla extract
- fruits to serve or a dollop of vegan whipped cream

Prep Time: 15 mins   **Serves:** 6
Cooking Time: 15 mins
Total Time: 30 mins

Instructions:

- In a small bowl/measuring cup, combine the nut milk, vanilla essence, and lemon juice or ACV. Allow for around 5 minutes to prepare the vegan buttermilk.
- Sift together the flour, baking powder, and salt in a large mixing bowl. The sifting contributes significantly to the airy texture of the waffles.
- Add the sugar, melted butter/oil, and buttermilk combination to the dry ingredients and gently fold together with a spatula until just incorporated. It is OK (and perhaps natural) to have some lumps. The batter should be thick but not too thick to scoop.

- Turn on and preheat your waffle maker to the desired oven temperature. I set mine to medium because I want my cookies crisp and brown but also fluffy.

- Scoop out some batter using a ½ cup (125mL) measuring cup and pour/spread it into the center of the greased waffle machine. You don't have to push it all the way to the edges. Close and leave to cook until the steam from the waffle maker has completely stopped. Don't open it till the steam is gone!

- Remove each waffle and keep warm and crispy on a baking sheet in your oven or toaster oven set to "warm" or 200F/95C until you've finished the entire batter. Continue with the remaining batter.

- Enjoy with your favorite toppings, such as blueberry sauce!

Nutritional Value

- Calories: 259kcal
- Carbohydrate: 36g
- Fats: 10g
- Protein: 6g

13. Almond Butter and Banana Toast

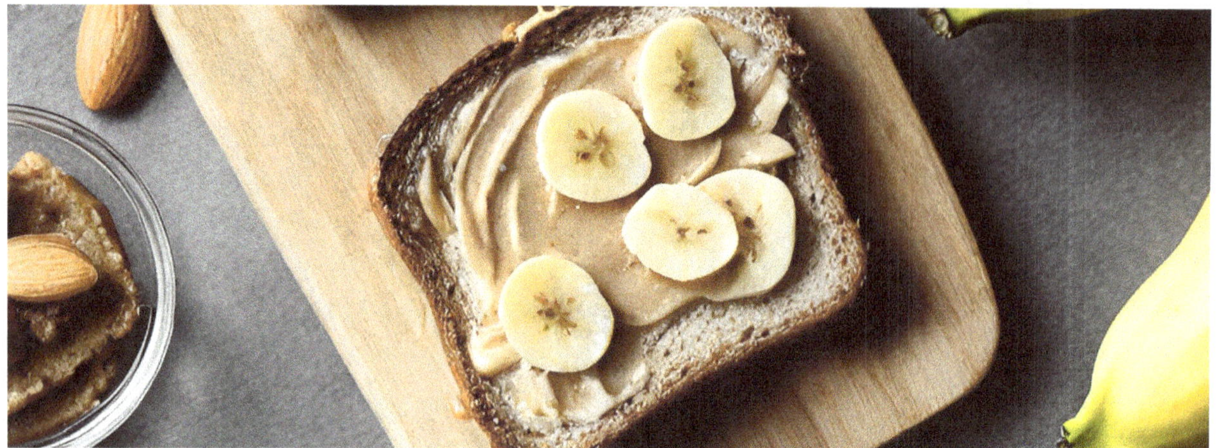

Ingredients:

- 1 tbsp. almond butter
- 1 toasted piece rye bread
- 1 sliced banana

Prep Time: 15 mins   **Serves:** 6

Cooking Time: 15 mins

Total Time: 30 mins

Instructions:

- Put the almond toast all over toas
- Top bread with almond butter.

Nutritional Value

- Calories: 280kcal
- Carbohydrate: 44g
- Fats: 11g
- Protein: 6g

14. Gluten-free Banana Pancakes

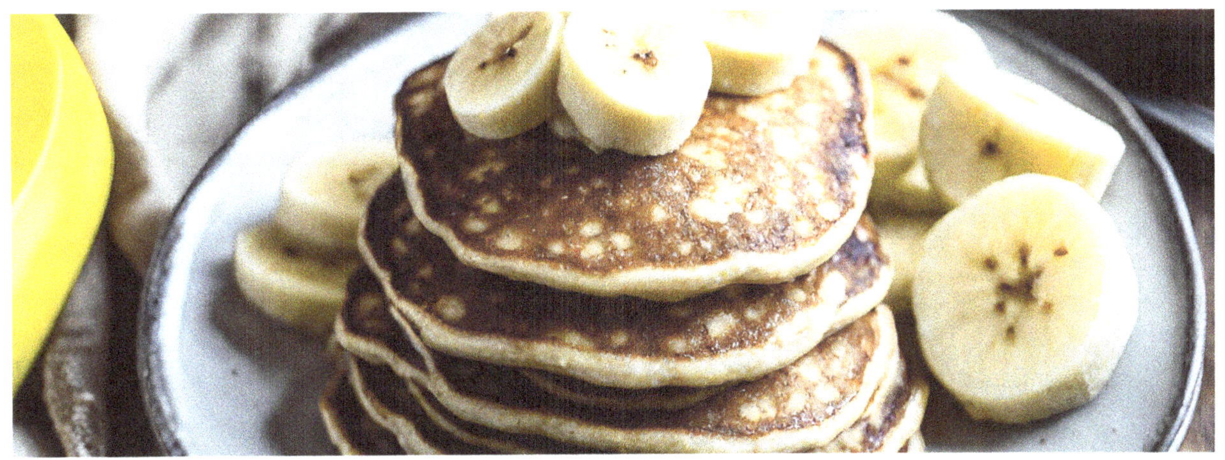

Ingredients:

- ¾ cup (75 g) gluten-free oat flour
  34 teaspoon baking powder
- a pinch of kosher salt
- 3 (150 g (weighed out of shell))
  room temperature eggs, well
  beaten
- 1½ (150 g) peeled, ripe banana,
  mashed

Prep Time: 10 mins **Serves:** 6
Cooking Time: 10 mins
Total Time: 20 mins

Instructions:

- Place the ground oats (or equivalent), baking powder, and optional salt in a medium-size mixing bowl or measuring cup with a pour spout. Whisk everything together thoroughly.
- Whisk in the beaten eggs and mashed banana until the texture is consistent.
- Preheat a griddle to 350°F or a nonstick, heavy-bottom skillet to medium heat. Using a small amount of (optional) butter, grease the heating surface.
- Whisk the pancake batter again to ensure homogeneity, then spoon it into 1/4-cup sections onto the hot, buttered skillet. Allow the

- pancakes to cook for 2 minutes, or until golden brown on the underside.
- Flip the pancakes and cook for about 30 seconds, or until they are set. Repeat with the remaining batter in the skillet or griddle. Serve hot.
- Leftover pancakes can be carefully wrapped and refrigerated for up to 3 days or frozen for longer periods of time.
- Allow to defrost at room temperature before unwrapping and placing on foil. Before serving, lightly sprinkle with water and reheat in a 300°F oven or toaster oven until warm.

Nutritional Value (all 6)

- Calories: 677kcal
- Carbohydrate: 113.5g
- Fats: 32.5g
- Protein: 28g

15. Flourless Banana Muffins

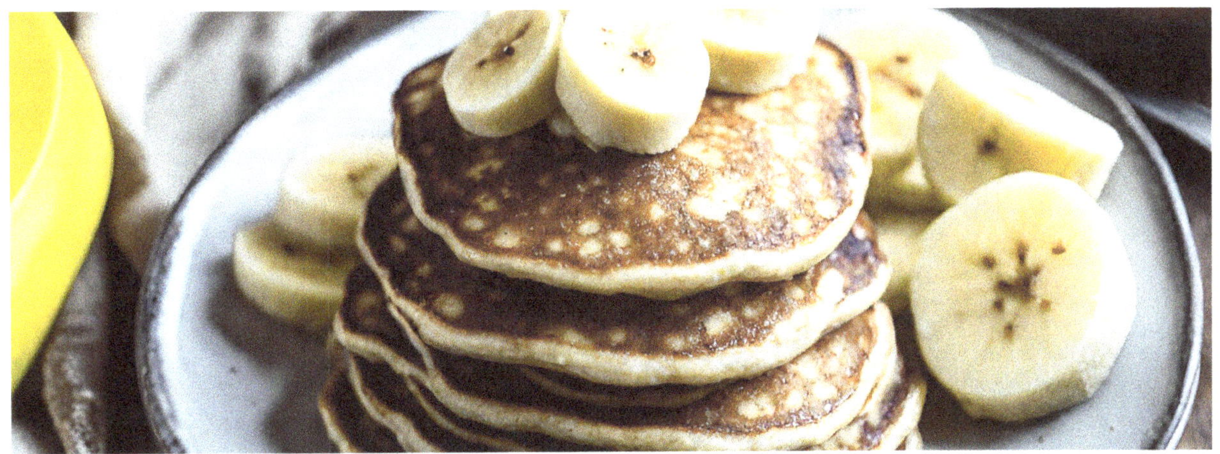

Ingredients:

- 2 cups quick or old-fashioned oats
- 3 very ripe bananas
- 2 eggs
- ¼ cup pure maple syrup
- 1 tsp. baking soda
- ¼ tsp kosher salt
- ¼ cup miniature chocolate chips

Prep Time: 5 mins

Cooking Time: 15 mins

Total Time: 20 mins

Serves: 12 muffins

Instructions:

- Preheat the oven to 350 degrees Fahrenheit. Line a muffin pan with paper liners or spray liberally with oil.
- Blend the oats in a blender. Blend for 30 seconds, or until the oats resemble flour in texture.
- In a blender, combine the peeled bananas, eggs, maple syrup, baking soda, and salt. Blend until a batter develops, scraping down the sides as necessary.
- Pulse the chocolate chips into the batter to evenly distribute them.
- Pour the batter into the muffin tray, dividing it evenly among the 12 muffins.
- When a toothpick put into the

- center comes out clean, bake for 15 to 17 minutes. These muffins keep best in the refrigerator after cooling, but they can also be frozen.

Nutritional Value (all 6)

- Calories: 677kcal
- Carbohydrate: 113.5g
- Fats: 32.5g
- Protein: 28g

Lunch Delights

16. Avocado and Lentil Power Bowl

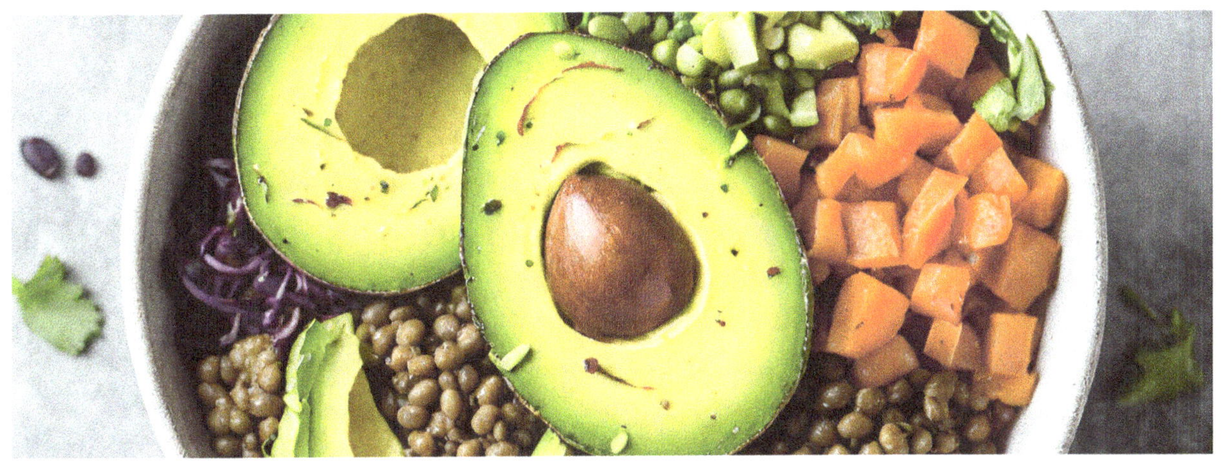

Ingredients:

- 1 medium cauliflower head, cut into florets
- 1 paprika teaspoon
- a half teaspoon garlic powder
- a half teaspoon onion powder
- season with salt & pepper
- 1 cup farro or other chosen grain (gluten-free if desired)
- 1 bunch chopped kale
- 1-2 minced garlic cloves
- 2 cups drained and rinsed black beans
- 1 pound sauerkraut
- For garnish, use sliced green onions or cilantro.

To make Avocado Pesto:
- a single avocado
- ¼ cup packed fresh basil

Instructions:

- Preheat the oven to 400 degrees Fahrenheit. Lightly oil a baking sheet.
- Arrange the cauliflower florets on a baking pan. Add salt, pepper, onion powder, garlic powder, and paprika to taste. To provide an even coating, stir. Bake the potatoes for 20 minutes, or until they are tender.
- In a medium pot, cook farro (or similar grain) as directed on the package. The cooked grains should be put in a basin.
- In the same saucepan, preheat

- Optional: a handful of spinach
- Juice of ½ lemon
- 2 garlic cloves
- 2 teaspoons walnuts

Prep Time: 10 mins   **Serves:** 4

Cooking Time: 20 mins

Total Time: 30 mins

- some water. Add the greens, salt, pepper, and garlic. Cook until the kale has wilted, about 5 minutes.
- Arrange kale, grains, beans, cauliflower, sauerkraut, avocado pesto, and fresh herbs in bowls.
- To make the avocado pesto, combine the avocado, basil, spinach, lemon juice, garlic, and walnuts in a blender or small food processor. If necessary, add a couple tablespoons of water and pulse until smooth.

Nutritional Value

- Calories: 400kcal
- Carbohydrate: 67.5g
- Fats: 8.8g
- Protein: 19.6mg

17. Broccoli And Cauliflower Rice Stir Fry

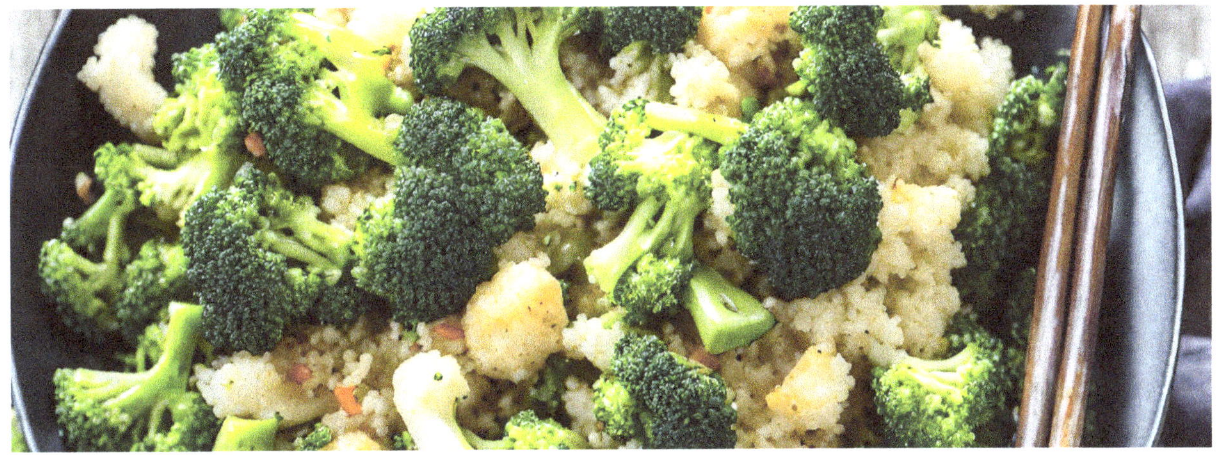

Ingredients:

- 1 medium cauliflower head, broken into florets
- ½ teaspoon sea salt, crushed
- ½ teaspoon black pepper, freshly ground
- ½ tsp garlic powder
- 2 tbsp. sesame oil
- 2 cups broccoli florets (cut into bite-sized pieces)
- 1 cup lightly chopped shredded carrots
- ½ cup finely sliced green onions
- 1 cup shelled fresh or frozen edamame (no need to thaw if frozen)
- Sauce
- 1 teaspoon dried ginger or 2 tablespoons minced ginger
- 2 tbsp. sesame oil
- 2 tbsp soy sauce (or tamari if gluten-free)
- two tbsp rice vinegar

Instructions:

- Combine the cauliflower florets, salt, pepper, and garlic powder in a food processor. Pulse for 20 to 30 seconds, or until the texture is coarse and similar to rice.
- To make the sauce, mix all sauce ingredients in a small bowl and whisk together.
- Heat 2 teaspoons of sesame oil in a large pot or wok over medium heat. Cook the broccoli and carrots for 4-5 minutes, stirring periodically, until the broccoli is tender.
- Cook for 3-4 minutes, stirring periodically, until the edamame and green onions are heated through. Set aside the vegetables from the skillet.

- ½ to 1 teaspoon Sriracha
- ½ tablespoon maple syrup or agave nectar
- 1 tbsp unsalted organic natural smooth smooth peanut butter

Prep Time: 10 mins   **Serves:** 4

Cooking Time: 10 mins

Total Time: 20 mins

- Cook the cauliflower in the skillet for 4-5 minutes, or until it is tender. Remove from the heat and toss in the vegetables and sauce. Serve with a stir.
- Refrigerate in an airtight container. This meal is best served immediately, but it can be stored in the refrigerator for up to 2-3 days.

Nutritional Value

- Calories: 400kcal
- Carbohydrate: 67.5g
- Fats: 8.8g
- Protein: 19.6mg

18. Vegetable Frittata

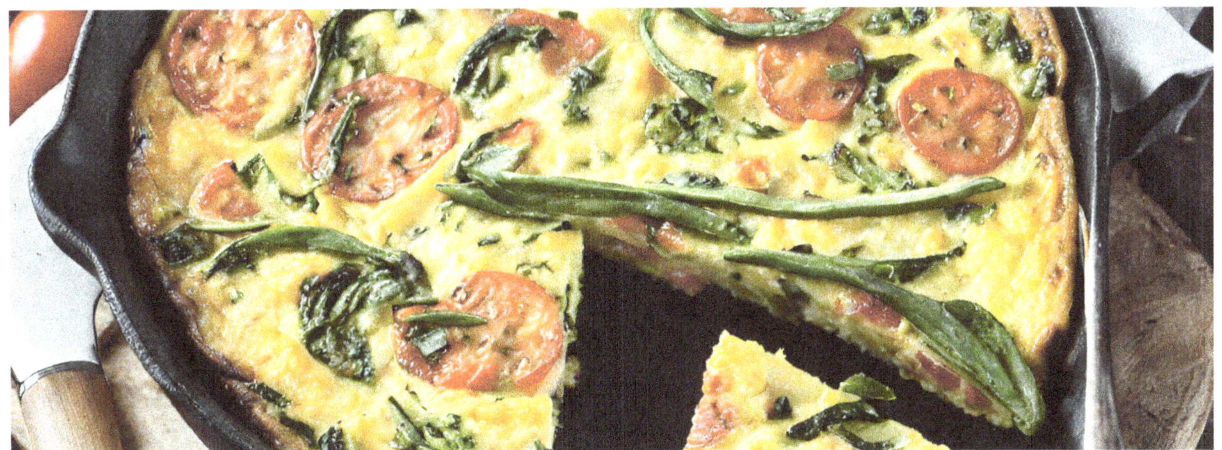

Ingredients:

- 6 eggs
- ¼ cup yogurt (whole milk)
- ¼ cup chopped red onions
- 1 cup of divided shredded mozzarella cheese
- ¼ cup cilantro chopped
- ½ cup cherry tomatoes sliced
- 1 cup mushrooms chopped
- 8-10 stalks asparagus ends cut and chopped

Instructions:

- Preheat the oven to 425° degrees.
- Set aside the egg, yogurt, half of the shredded mozzarella cheese, and salt and pepper.
- In an oven-safe or cast-iron pan, heat the olive oil. Cook for 3-5 minutes, or until the onions, mushrooms, and asparagus soften.
- Place the cooked vegetables on top of the egg mixture. Top with the remaining cheese and cut cherry tomatoes.
- Bake uncovered in a preheated oven for 10-15 minutes, or until the middle is firm and not jiggly.

Prep Time: 10 mins   **Serves:** 4
Cooking Time: 15 mins
Total Time: 25 mins

Nutritional Value

- Calories: 216 kcal
- Carbohydrate: 6g
- Fats: 11g
- Protein: 17mg

19. Chilled Tomato Gazpacho Soup

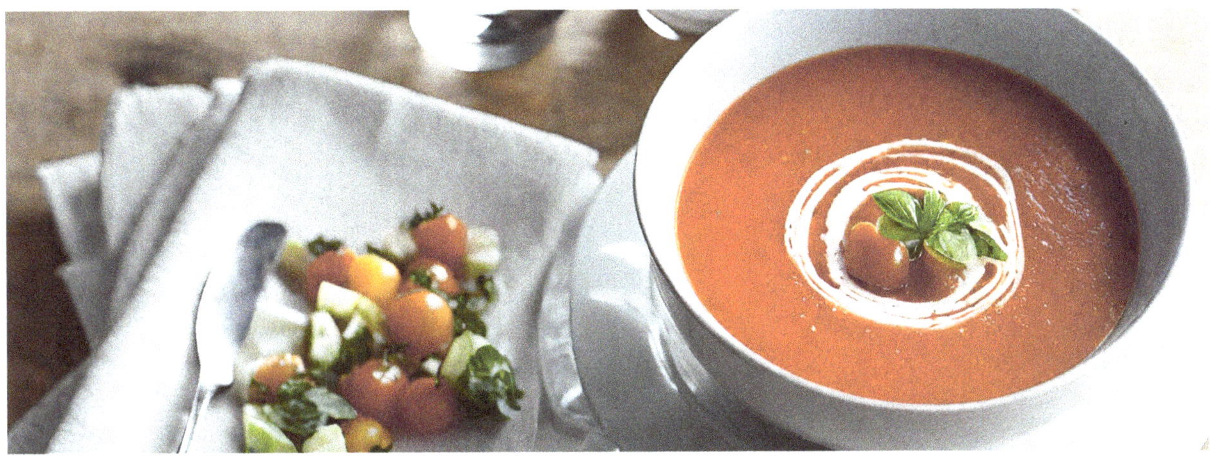

Ingredients:

- 2 big peeled tomatoes
- 1 large peeled and halved cucumber
- 1 peeled and halved onion
- 1 green bell pepper, seeded and quartered
- ¼ cup extra-virgin olive oil, split
- 24 oz. divided tomato juice
- ⅓ cup vinegar (red wine)
- ¼ teaspoon black pepper
- ½ teaspoon kosher salt
- a few squirts of spicy sauce
- ¼ cup coarsely chopped chives
- 1 garlic clove, minced

Prep Time: 15 mins   **Serves:** 4

Addit. Time: 2 hrs

Total Time: 2hrs 15mins

Instructions:

- In a blender, combine 1 tomato, ½ cucumber, ½ onion, ¼ bell pepper, and ½ cup tomato juice until smooth.
- Transfer to a mixing bowl and stir in the remaining tomato juice, olive oil, vinegar, salt, pepper, and spicy sauce.
- Before serving, make sure to refrigerate for at least 2 hours.
- Refrigerate the leftover vegetables separately from the soup.
- Before serving, add the garlic and diced vegetables. Serve chilled, topped with chives.
- Leftovers can be stored in the fridge for up to 5 days.

- Calories: 134 kcal
- Carbohydrate: 12g
- Fats: 10g
- Protein: 2g

20. Sweet Potato Vegan Buddha Bowl

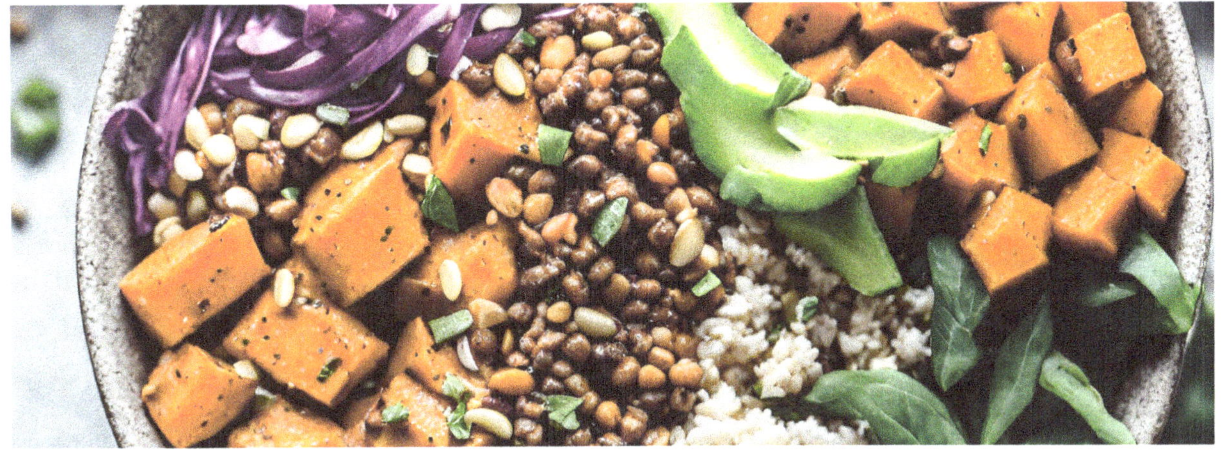

Ingredients:

- Roasted Sweet potatoes
  - 1 tablespoon olive oil
  - 3 big diced sweet potatoes
  - ½ teaspoon garlic powder
  - 1/2 teaspoon salt
- Cubes of roasted tofu
  - 1 container drained and pressed firm tofu
  - 1 teaspoon of olive oil
  - a half teaspoon garlic powder
  - ¼ teaspoon black pepper
  - ¼ teaspoon salt
- Kale, Shredded
- Cooked Avocado Couscous or other desired grain
- Avocado slices with seeds for garnish
- Tahini Lemon Dressing
  - ⅓ cup tahini
  - ¼ teaspoon lemon juice
  - ½ teaspoon salt

Instructions:

- Preheat the oven to 400 degrees Fahrenheit.
- To make the sweet potatoes, follow these steps: Toss the sweet potatoes with the olive oil, garlic, salt, and pepper. Place on a baking sheet in a single layer and tent loosely with foil. Cook for 20 minutes, then remove the foil and continue to cook for another 15-20 minutes, or until crispy.
- To prepare the tofu: Toss the tofu in a bowl with the olive oil, garlic powder, salt, and pepper. Cook for 20 minutes, until golden brown and crispy, on a separate baking sheet in a single layer.
- Cook the couscous and slice the

- 2 large garlic cloves, minced
- ¼ cup cold water
- 1 pinch ground cumin

Prep Time: 20 mins   **Serves:** 4
Cooking Time: 40 mins
Total Time: 60 mins

Nutritional Value

- Calories: 312 kcal
- Carbohydrate: 51g
- Fats: 10g
- Protein: 10mg

- kale while the potatoes and tofu are cooking.
- To make the lemon tahini dressing, follow these steps: In a mixing bowl, combine the tahini, lemon juice, garlic, salt, and cumin. Add the water a spoonful at a time, whisking constantly, until the mixture is creamy; it may likely seize up on you, but don't worry, just keep whisking. Continue to add water until the mixture is creamy and smooth.
- Assemble! Divide the couscous, sweet potatoes, kale, and tofu among four bowls; sprinkle with lemon tahini sauce and top with avocado and your favorite nuts/seeds.

21. Salmon With Green Bean Almondine

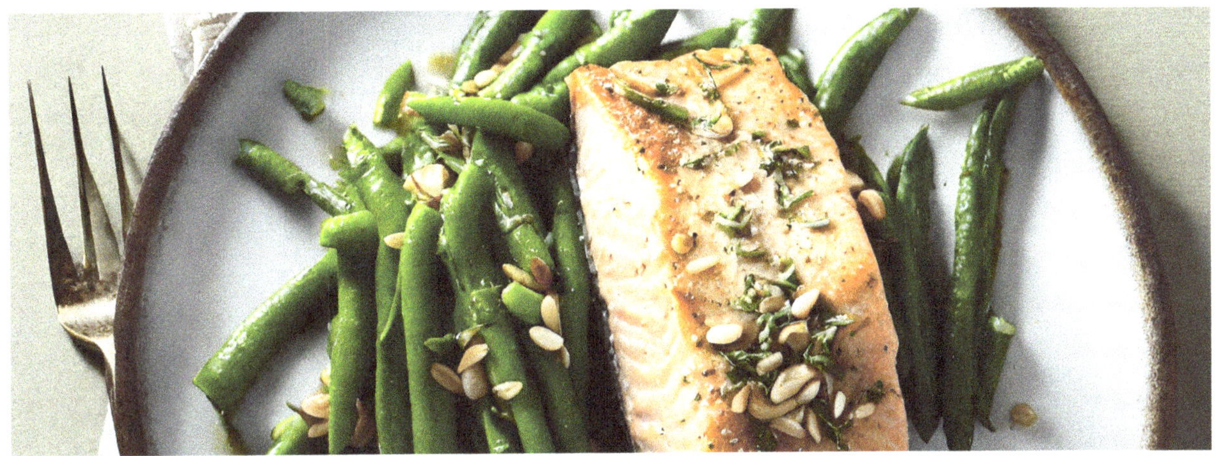

Ingredients:

- Tablespoon of Heinz Dijon Mustard
- ¼ cup Kraft Extra Virgin Olive Oil Aged Balsamic Vinaigrette Dressing, divided
- 1½ tsp chopped garlic, divided skinless salmon filets (1 pound/450 g)
- 1 lb (450 g) fresh green beans, trimmed
- ¼ cup toasted sliced almonds

Prep Time: 20 mins   **Serves:** 4

Cooking Time: 20 mins

Total Time: 40 mins

Instructions:

- Preheat the broiler.
- Place the fish on a broiler pan rack sprayed with cooking spray. Spread mustard, 1 tablespoon dressing, and ½ teaspoon garlic on top of the fish.
- Broil for 6 to 8 minutes, 4 inches from the fire, or until the salmon flakes easily with a fork. In the meantime, place the beans in a medium pot and cover with water.
- Bring to a boil, then reduce to a medium-low heat for 6 minutes, or until the beans are crisp-tender. In a colander, drain the beans.
- Cook for 1 minute over medium heat, stirring regularly, with the remaining dressing and garlic. Cook for 2 minutes, stirring

- regularly, after adding the beans. Finish with nuts.
- Serve alongside seafood.

Nutritional Value

- Calories: 250 kcal
- Carbohydrate: 11g
- Fats: 12g
- Protein: 25g

22. Grilled Lemon Herb Chicken Salad

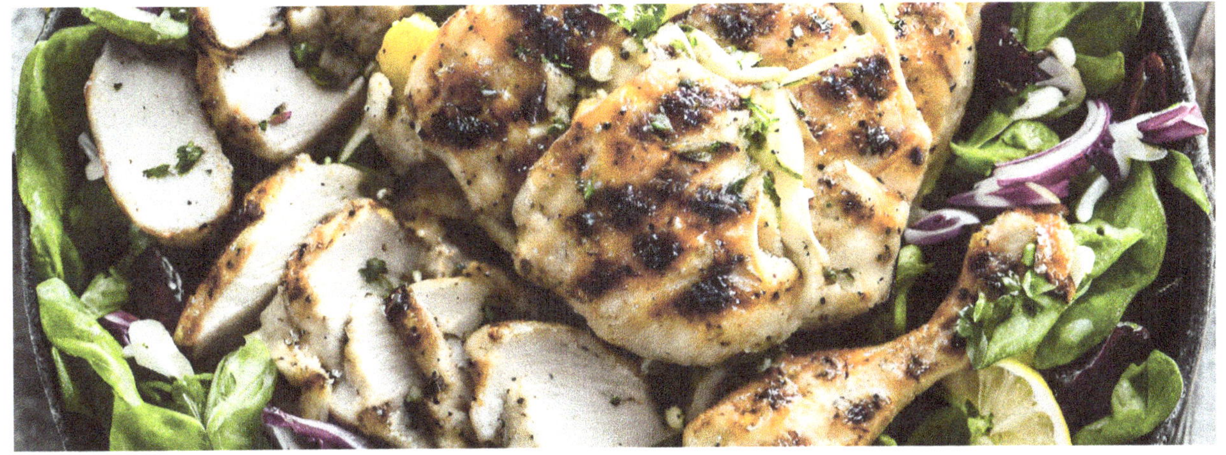

Ingredients:

Marinade/Dressing:
- 1 lemon juice (¼ cup fresh squeezed)
- 2 teaspoons olive oil
- 2 teaspoons water
- 2 tbsp of red wine vinegar
- 2 tbsp freshly chopped parsley
- 2 tablespoons dried basil
- 2 teaspoons minced garlic
- 1 tsp. dried oregano
- 1 tsp salt and cracked pepper, to taste
- 1 pound (500 g) skinless, boneless chicken thigh filets

Salad:
- 4 cups washed and dried Romaine (or Cos) lettuce leaves
- 1 big sliced cucumber
- 2 diced Roma tomatoes
- 1 sliced red onion
- 1 sliced avocado

Instructions:

- In a large mixing bowl, combine all of the marinade/dressing ingredients. Half of the marinade should be poured into a big, shallow dish. Refrigerate any leftover marinade to use as a dressing later.
- Add the chicken to the bowl and marinate for 15-30 minutes (or up to two hours in the refrigerator if time allows). While you wait for the chicken, prepare the salad ingredients and combine them in a big salad dish.
- Heat 1 tablespoon of oil in a grill pan or grill plate over medium-high heat once the chicken is done. Grill the chicken on both sides

- (optional) ⅓ cup pitted and sliced Kalamata olives (or black olives)
- Serve with lemon wedges

Prep Time: 10 mins   **Serves:** 4
Cooking Time: 15 mins
Total Time: 25 mins

Nutritional Value

- Calories: 336 kcal
- Carbohydrate: 13g
- Fats: 21g
- Protein: 24g

- until it is browned and cooked through.
- Allow chicken to rest for 5 minutes before slicing and serving over salad. Drizzle the leftover UNTOUCHED dressing over the salad. With lemon slices, serve.

23. Banana Nut Muffins

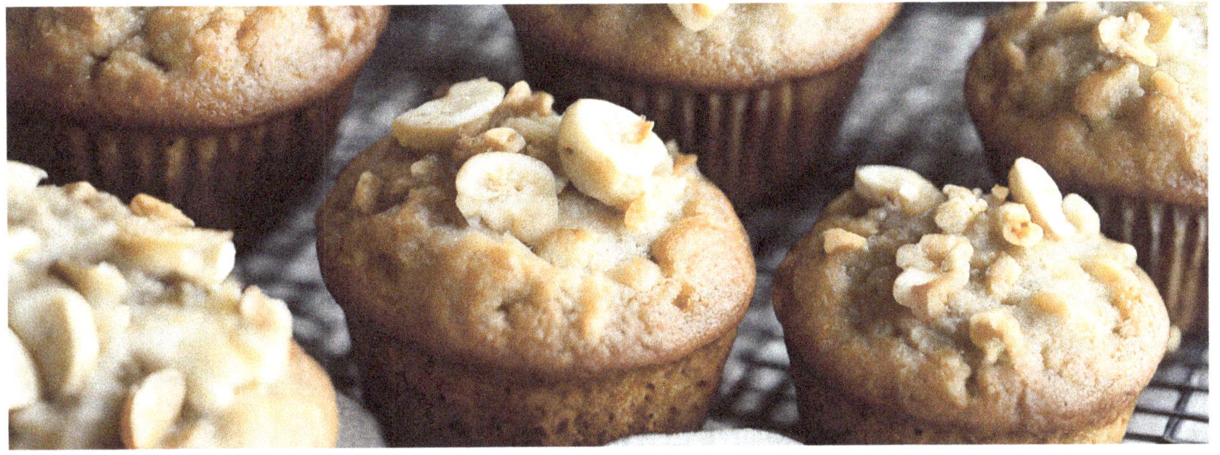

Ingredients:

Instructions:

Muffins
- 0.33 cup unsalted butter, melted and gently cooled
- 0.44 cup light brown sugar, lightly packed (fresh and soft).
- 1.33 big eggs
- 1.33 cup mashed very ripe bananas (about 3-4 bananas)
- 1.17 cup all-purpose flour
- 1.33 teaspoon pure vanilla extract
- 1 teaspoon baking soda
- Optional: 0.17 teaspoon salt and 0.33 teaspoon ground cinnamon
- 0.33 cup chopped walnuts, or substitute macadamia, pecan, or hazelnuts

Topping:
- 0.17 cup granulated sugar
- 1.33 to 2 tbsp. chopped walnuts

- Preheat the oven to 350 degrees Fahrenheit.
- In a large mixing bowl, whisk together melted butter and 23 cup brown sugar for 1 minute. Whisk in the eggs, mashed banana, and vanilla extract until well blended.
- Combine the flour, baking soda, salt, and cinnamon in a separate bowl.
- Add the dry ingredients to the wet components and whisk with a rubber spatula until almost incorporated. Stir in ½ cup chopped nuts until no flour streaks remain. Take care not to over-mix.
- Grease 15 standard-sized muffin

Prep Time: 15 mins   **Serves:** 10

Cooking Time: 15 mins

Total Time: 30 mins

Nutritional Value

- Calories: 231kcal
- Carbohydrate: 32g
- Fats: 10g
- Protein: 3g

- cups and distribute the batter evenly.
- Topping: Sprinkle brown sugar and chopped walnuts on top of each cup. A toothpick put into the center should come out clean after 14–17 minutes. Place the pan on a wire rack to cool.

24. Spinach and Turkey Stuffed Peppers

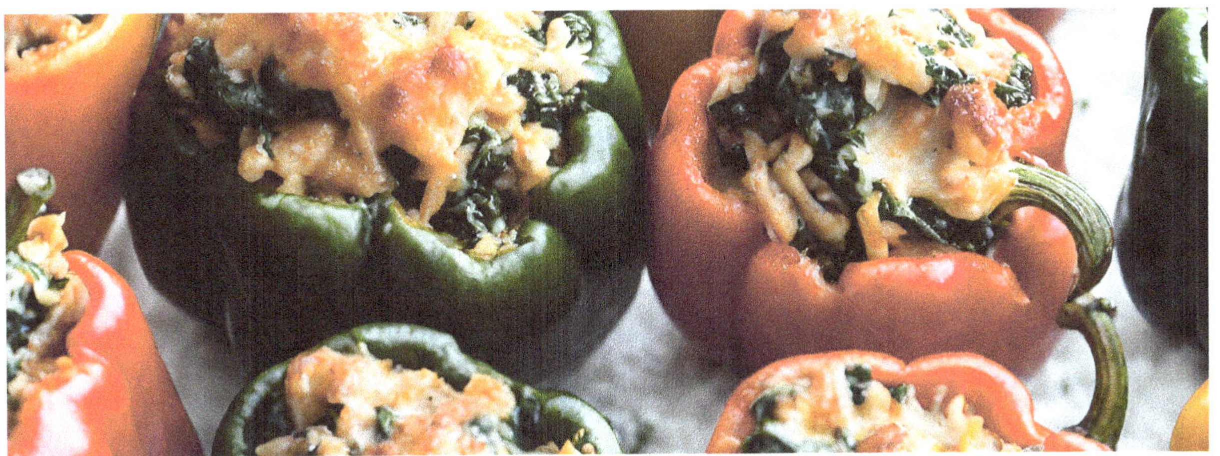

Ingredients:

- 4 green bell peppers, trimmed and seeded
- 2 teaspoons olive oil
- 1 pound ground turkey
- 2 tbsp olive oil
- ½ chopped onion
- ½ onion, diced
- 1 cup sliced mushrooms
- ½ red bell pepper, diced
- ½ yellow bell pepper, chopped
- 1 zucchini, chopped
- ½ red bell pepper, chopped
- ½ yellow bell pepper, chopped
- 1 cup fresh spinach
- 1 (14.5 oz) can chopped tomatoes, drained
- 1 tbsp tomato paste
- Italian seasoning to taste
- Garlic powder to taste
- Salt and pepper to taste

Instructions:

- Preheat the oven to 350°F (175°C).
- Collect all of the components.
- Wrap green bell peppers in aluminum foil and set in a baking dish. Bake for 15 minutes in a preheated oven. Remove from the oven.
- Cook the turkey in a pan over medium heat until it is evenly browned. Set aside.
- In a skillet, heat the oil and sauté the onion, mushrooms, zucchini, red bell pepper, yellow bell pepper, and spinach until soft. Return the turkey to the skillet. Season with Italian seasoning, garlic powder, salt, and pepper

Prep Time: 20 mins   **Serves:** 4

Cooking Time: 40 mins

Total Time: 60 mins

Nutritional Value

- Calories: 279kcal
- Carbohydrate: 10g
- Fats: 16g
- Protein: 25g

- after adding the tomatoes and tomato paste. Place the skillet mixture inside the green peppers.
- After 15 minutes, put the peppers back in the oven to continue baking.
- Serve hot and enjoy.

25. Veggie-Packed Shrimp Spring Rolls

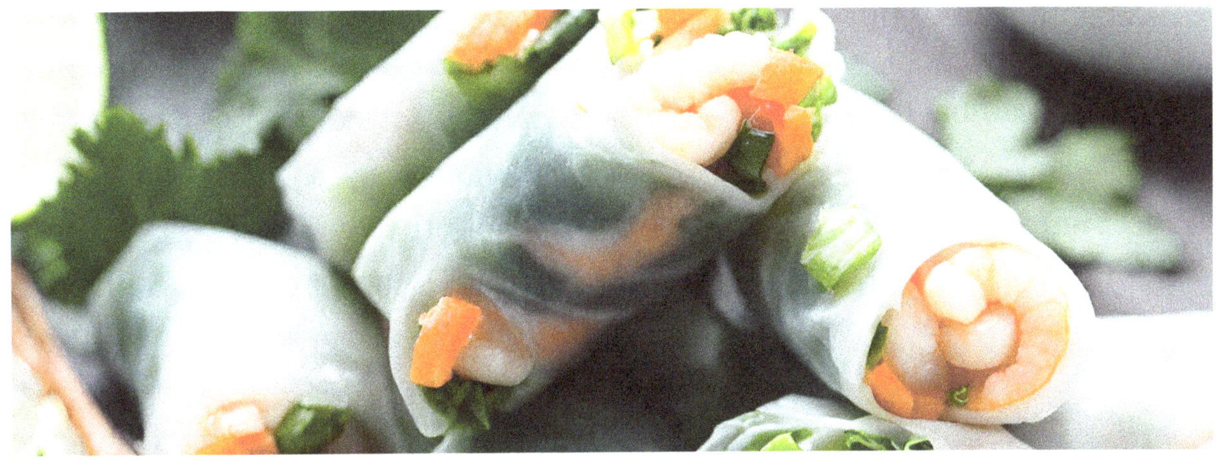

Ingredients:

- a dozen to fifteen rice paper wrappers
- 1 romaine lettuce head, with leaves separated and the largest leaves cut in half
- I used roughly 4 ounces of uncooked vermicelli noodles.
- 1 pound cooked shrimp, shells and tails removed (whole or halves)
- ½ cucumber, cut into matchsticks
- 1 medium carrot, cut into matchsticks
- 1 sliced avocado (optional)
- mint or fresh basil

Peanut Sauce
- 14 oz. peanut butter
- 1-2 tablespoons coconut milk, regular or light
- 1 garlic clove, sliced
- 2 tablespoons fresh ginger, chopped.

Instructions:

- Cook the vermicelli noodles according per the package directions. Rinse with cold water after draining. Place aside.
- To make the dipping sauce, mix all of the ingredients in a blender and blend until smooth, starting with 1 tablespoon of coconut milk and adding more as needed to achieve the desired consistency.
- Warm the water in a pot over the stove. You only want warm water, not boiling water. Pour heated water into a dish or plate large enough to hold the rice paper wrappers. A pie plate works great! Dip rice paper wrappers in warm water for 15-20 seconds, or until

- 2 teaspoons rice vinegar
- 2 tbsp tamari, soy sauce, or coconut aminos (low sodium)
- 2 teaspoons maple syrup
- 1-2 tsp. sambal oelek

Prep Time: 35 mins   **Serves:** 4
Cooking Time: 0 mins
Total Time: 35 mins

Nutritional Value

- Calories: 282 kcal
- Carbohydrate: 33g
- Fats: 10g
- Protein: 15g

- they soften somewhat. Allowing papers to soak in water for too long may cause them to become overly soft and floppy, causing them to tear as you roll.
- Place the wrapper on a firm surface, such as a plate. Place a lettuce leaf on the wrapper's far left border. Place a few pieces of each item into the lettuce leaf, roughly 3-4 pieces of shrimp, carrots, cucumbers, and noodles. Top with 1 avocado slice (if using) and fresh herbs.
- Roll the wrapper from left to right, folding the top and bottom sides toward the center (like an envelope) approximately midway through wrapping.
- Steps 1–4 must be completed for each wrapper. Serve with the peanut sauce on the side.

26. Eggplant Parmesan Stacks

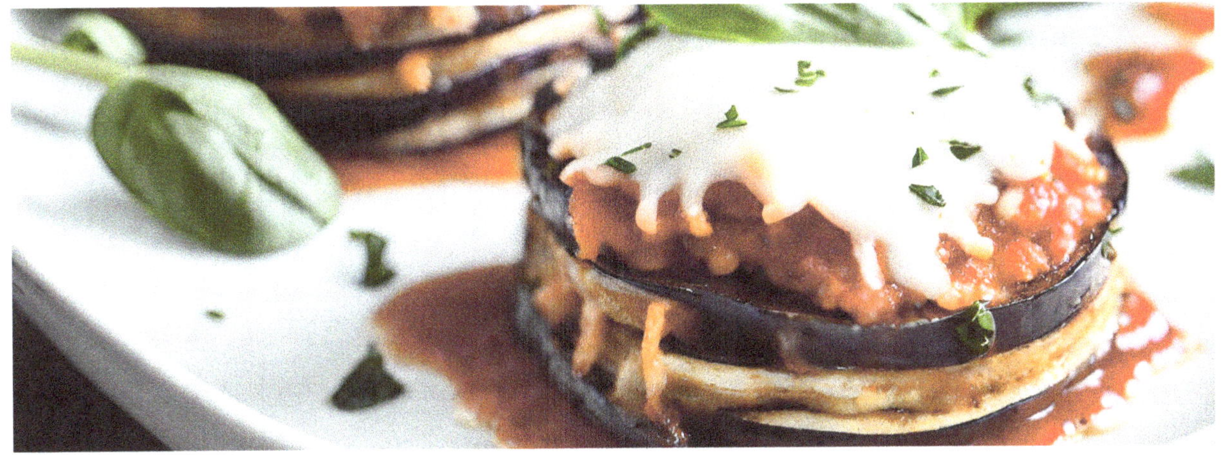

Ingredients:

- 2 medium eggplants, cut into ½-inch rounds
- 1 tsp salt to extract moisture from the eggplant
- A pinch of salt and pepper to taste
- 4 eggs
- 4 cups bread crumbs (panko)
- 1 cooking spray
- 1 jar RAG® Old World Style® Traditional Sauce (24 oz.)
- 2 (8 ounce) packages finely sliced mozzarella cheese
- 1 cup parmesan cheese, grated.

Instructions:

- Preheat the oven to 425 degrees Fahrenheit (220 degrees Celsius).
- Sprinkle salt on both sides of the eggplant rounds and lay on a baking sheet for 15 minutes to suck out moisture. Blot the liquid from either side of the eggplant slices with paper towels. To taste, add salt and pepper for seasoning.
- Whisk the eggs in a small dish. Mix the panko bread crumbs in another basin. Dip each side of the eggplant slices into the whisked eggs, then coat with panko crumbs. Place the slices on a baking sheet with a cooling rack.
- Coat the tops of the eggplant with cooking spray. In a preheated

Prep Time: 20 mins   **Serves:** 4

Cooking Time: 40 mins

Total Time: 60 mins

Nutritional Value

- Calories: 239kcal
- Carbohydrate: 50g
- Fats: 16g
- Protein: 15g

- oven, bake for 8 minutes. Spray the other side of each slice with cooking spray. Bake for another 8 to 10 minutes. Allow to cool slightly after removing from the oven.
- Reduce the oven temperature to 350°F (175°C).
- To make the stacks, follow these steps: Use parchment paper to line a baking sheet. Place a large slice of eggplant on a piece of parchment paper. A dollop of Ragu® Old World Style® Traditional Sauce and a piece of mozzarella complete the dish. Layer another slice of eggplant on top of the first; continue layering until you have around 5 or 6 slices in a stack. Add a liberal layer of parmesan cheese on top.
- Bake the stacks for 10 to 15 minutes, or until the cheese has melted. Remove from the oven and set aside for a few minutes to cool. Serve hot.

27. Balsamic Glazed Fish

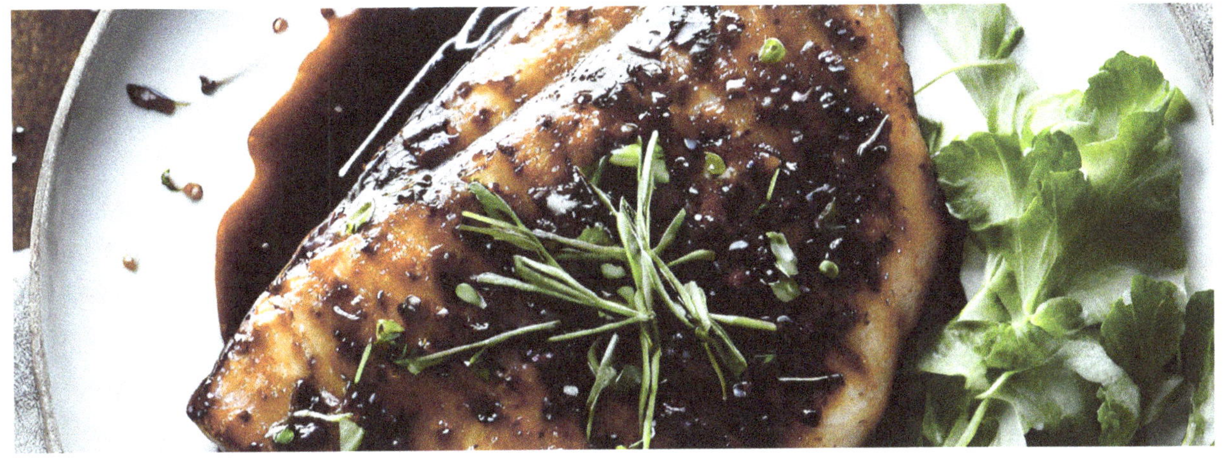

Ingredients:

- Four 5 oz. fish filets fish mahi mahi
- 1/2 teaspoon olive oil
- 1 tablespoon lemon juice
- ½ pound balsamic vinegar
- 2 teaspoon honey
- 1 tablespoon white wine
- 2 cloves garlic
- pepper, as desired

Prep Time: 10 mins   **Serves:** 4

Cooking Time: 20 mins

Total Time: 30 mins

Nutritional Value

- Calories: 194kcal
- Carbohydrate: 9g
- Fats: 4g
- Protein: 29g

Instructions:

- Preheat the oven to 400°F.
- Season the fish with salt and pepper. Place the fish in a casserole dish or on a baking sheet with sides to catch any juices.
- Drizzle one teaspoon olive oil and fresh lemon juice over the fish.
- Bake for 20 minutes, or until the filets are flaky and the internal temperature reaches 145°F.
- Make the glaze while the fish is cooking. Bring the balsamic vinegar, honey, wine, and garlic to a boil in a saucepan.
- Reduce the heat and simmer for 10-15 minutes, or until the sauce has thickened and decreased.
- Remove the fish from the oven,

- drizzle with balsamic glaze, and serve immediately.

28. Greek Quesadillas

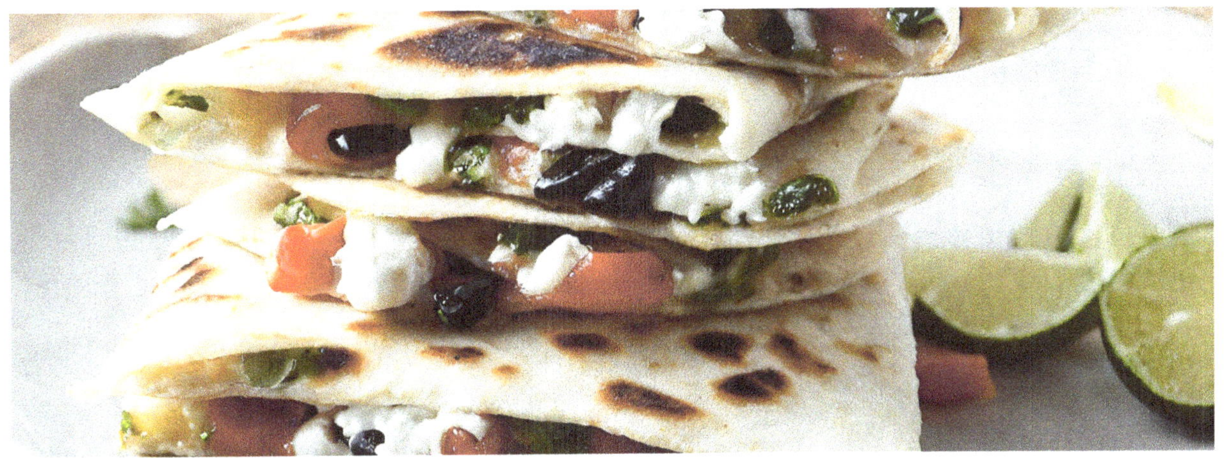

Ingredients:

Quesadillas

- 8 flour tortillas (8 inch)
- 1/2 cup chopped kalamata olives
- 1/2 cup drained and diced roasted red peppers
- 1 cup Feta cheese, crumbled
- 2 cups chicken shredded
- 3 cups shredded mozzarella
- Fresh dill shredded - chopped

Tzatziki

- 1 cup Greek yogurt, plain
- 1/2 cup finely sliced cucumber
- 1 tablespoon minced fresh dill 2 teaspoon lemon juice
- To taste, a teaspoon of salt and freshly cracked black pepper

Instructions:

Tzatziki

- In a small mixing dish, combine the Greek yogurt, cucumber, dill, and lemon juice. Season with salt and pepper to taste. Refrigerate while you prepare the quesadillas. This will allow the flavors to mingle in the sauce.

Quesadillas

- Preheat the oven to 400 degrees Fahrenheit. Line a baking sheet using a parchment paper
- Place two tortillas on the baking pan (my baking sheet only has room for two). Top with mozzarella, olives, red peppers, feta cheese, chicken, and a little more mozzarella, then finish with

Prep Time: 10 mins   **Serves:** 4

Cooking Time: 8 mins

Total Time: 18 mins

Nutritional Value

- Calories: 534 kcal
- Carbohydrate: 94g
- Fats: 34g
- Protein: 47g

- fresh chopped dill. Place another tortilla on top. Continue making quesadillas until you've created four.
- Bake for 8-10 minutes, or until the cheese is completely melted.
- Place the quesadilla on a platter and cut it in quarters. Serve right away with the tzatziki sauce.

29. Lean Turkey Paprikash

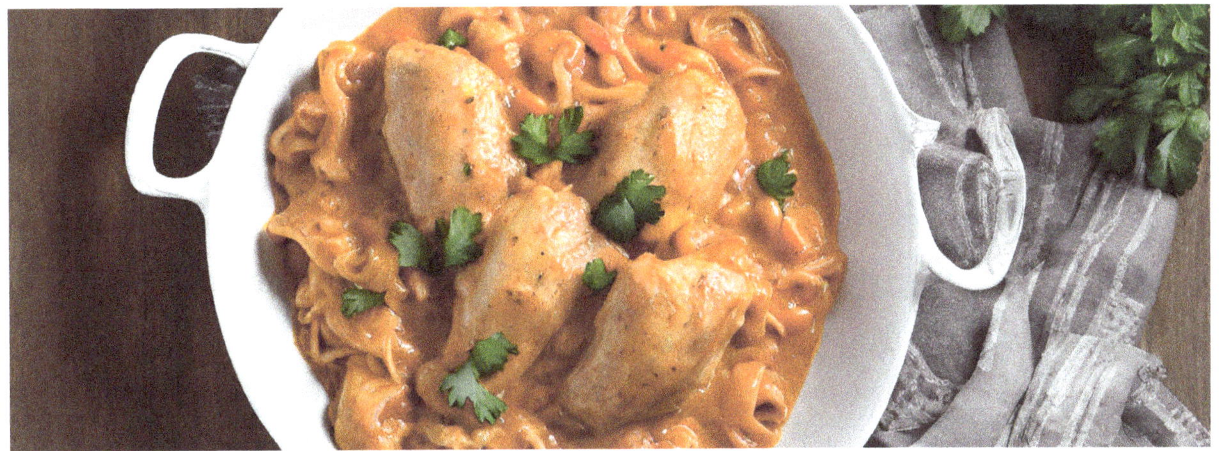

Ingredients:

- 1 pound ground turkey
- 1 big coarsely chopped onion
- 2 minced garlic cloves
- 1 chopped red bell pepper
- 1 chopped yellow bell pepper
- 1 tbsp. sweet paprika
- 1 smoked paprika teaspoon
- 1 tsp. caraway seeds
- 1 can (14 oz) undrained diced tomatoes
- 1 cup chicken broth (low sodium)
- Season with salt and pepper to taste.
- 1 cup plain Greek yogurt (serving size)
- chopped fresh parsley (for garnish)
- (Optional, for serving) whole-grain rice or quinoa

Instructions:

- Brown the lean ground turkey in a large skillet over medium heat until cooked through. Get rid of any extra fat.
- Sauté the chopped onions in the skillet until they are transparent.
- Add the minced garlic, sweet paprika, smoked paprika, and ground caraway seeds and mix well. Cook for a further 2 minutes to allow flavors to emerge.
- Pour in the diced tomatoes (with juice) and the chicken broth. To blend, stir everything together thoroughly.
- To the skillet, add sliced red and green bell peppers. Season to taste with salt and pepper. Cook for

Prep Time: 15 mins   **Serves:** 4
Cooking Time: 25 mins
Total Time: 40 mins

Nutritional Value

- Calories: 340 kcal
- Carbohydrate: 15g
- Fats: 16g
- Protein: 32g

- 15-20 minutes, or until the peppers are cooked.
- Prepare a bed of cauliflower rice or whole-grain rice for dishing while the sauce simmers.
- Taste and adjust seasoning as needed once the peppers are tender.
- Serve the turkey paprikash with cauliflower rice or whole-grain rice on the side. Garnish each plate with a dollop of plain Greek yogurt and fresh parsley.

30. Honey Orange Glazed Chicken

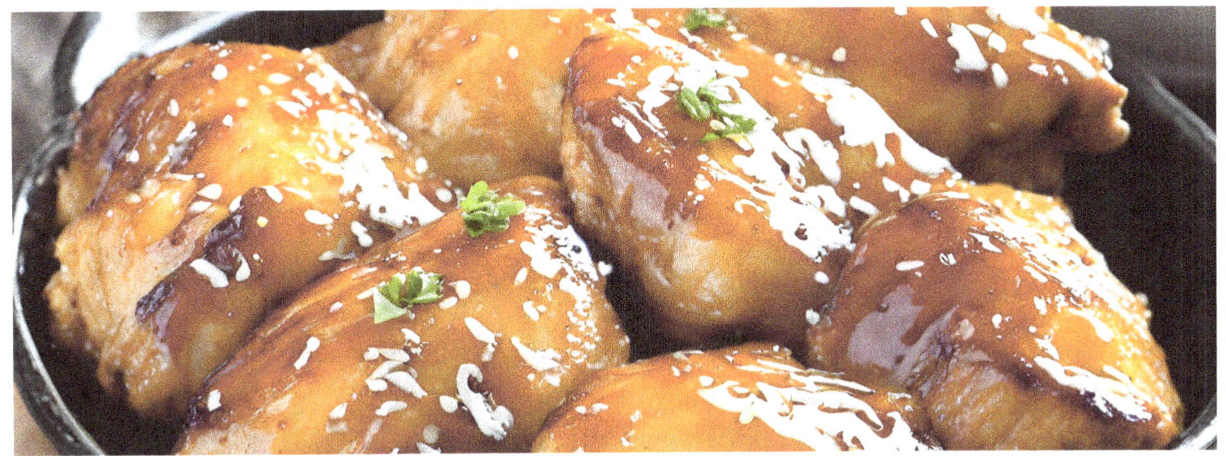

Ingredients:

- 1 glass orange juice
- ½ cup apple cider vinegar
- ½ cup packed brown sugar
- ¼ cup honey
- 1 teaspoon chili powder
- 1 teaspoon coriander powder
- 1 tablespoon cumin powder
- 2 lbs chicken thighs
- 1 tbsp olive oil
- salt and pepper

Prep Time: 5 mins   **Serves:** 6

Cooking Time: 45 mins

Total Time: 50 mins

Nutritional Value

- Calories: 501 kcal
- Carbohydrate: 37g
- Fats: 28g
- Protein: 26g

Instructions:

- Combine orange juice, cider vinegar, brown sugar, honey, chili powder, coriander, and cumin in a small pot. Bring to a boil, then reduce to a low heat and continue to cook for 35-45 minutes, or until the sauce has reduced to one cup.
- Heat the olive oil in a medium saucepan over medium high heat. Season the chicken thighs with salt and pepper and cook until the middle is 165°F and no longer pink. Drizzle the glaze over the top and allow it to simmer for 1-2 minutes, making sure the chicken is fully coated. Serve right away.

Dinner Recipes

31. Pan Seared Salmon

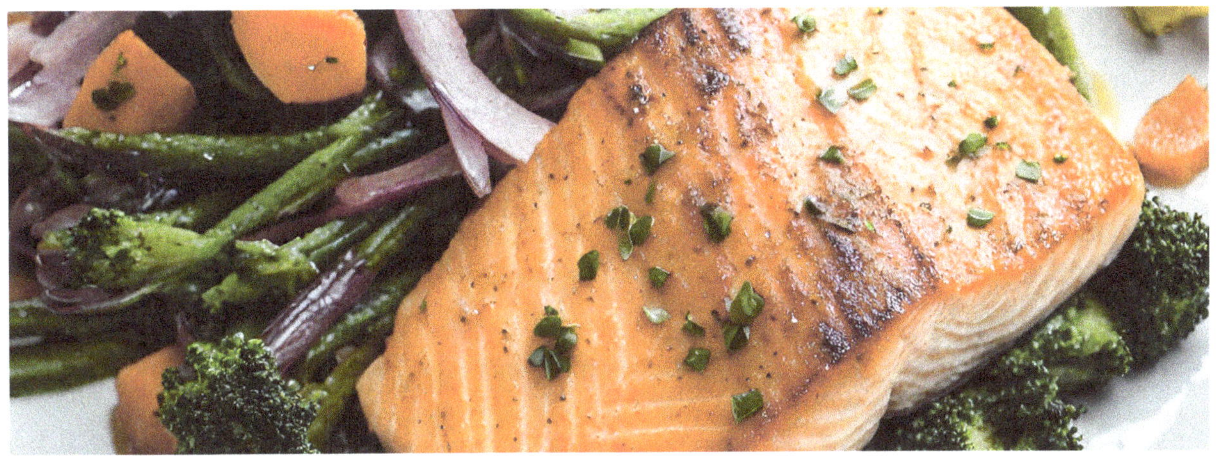

Ingredients:

- 4 (6–8-ounce) salmon filets, skin
- Half a teaspoon of kosher salt plus a few pinches
- ¼ teaspoon black pepper, ground
- 1 tbsp. unsalted butter
- ½ tablespoon high-smoke-point cooking oil (canola, grapeseed, avocado, or other)
- 1 lemon, peeled and cut into wedges
- Optional serving garnishes: chopped fresh parsley, basil, or dill

Instructions:

- Remove the salmon from the refrigerator and let aside for at least 10 minutes to come to room temperature. Pat the filets dry on both sides with a paper towel.
- In a 12-inch cast iron or heavy stainless steel skillet, heat the butter and oil over medium-high heat until the butter foams and the foam subsides, about 3 minutes. It is critical that the pan is very hot before adding the salmon, or it will not crisp properly.
- Season the flesh side of the salmon with 1/2 teaspoon salt and pepper

Prep Time: 10 mins   **Serves:** 4

Cooking Time: 15 mins

Total Time: 25 mins

Nutritional Value

- Calories: 290kcal
- Carbohydrate: 3g
- Fats: 34g
- Protein: 15g

- just before placing it to the skillet.
- Place the filets skin-side up in the skillet, lowering them away from you to protect yourself from splatters. Using a pinch of kosher salt, season the skin side of the salmon.
- Allow the salmon to cook on the first side entirely undisturbed for 5 to 6 minutes, or until the meat appears cooked approximately 3/4 of the way up the filet.
- Carefully flip the filets using a fish spatula or equivalent long, wide, flexible spatula. They should easily release from the pan; if they are stuck, the salmon is probably not cooked yet. Allow it to cook for another 30 seconds or so before attempting again.
- Reduce the heat in the pan to medium. Cook the fish for 2 to 4 minutes more on the other side, or until done to your preference (I remove the salmon at 130°F for medium). Transfer to a platter and let aside for 5 minutes. Sprinkle with herbs and squeeze lemon over the top. Serve immediately or at room temperature.

32. Pollo Fajitas

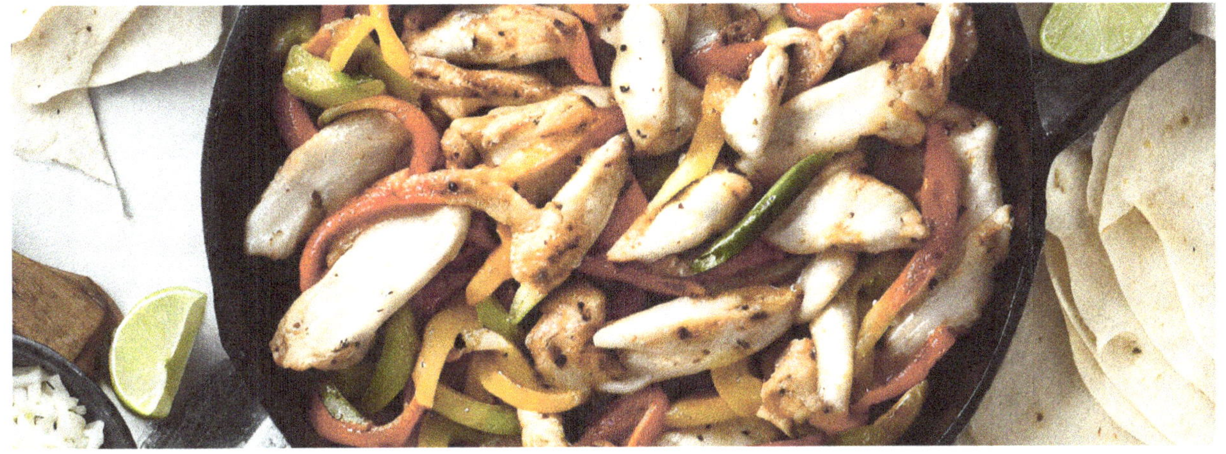

Ingredients:

- 1 tbsp. Worcestershire sauce
- 1 tbsp. cider vinegar
- 1 teaspoon of soy sauce
- 1 tsp. chili powder
- 1 minced garlic clove
- 1 teaspoon spicy pepper sauce
- 1½ pound boneless, skinless chicken thighs, sliced
- 1 tbsp. vegetable oil
- 1 finely sliced onion
- ½ lemon, juiced
- 1 green bell pepper, diced

Prep Time: 15 mins   **Serves:** 5

Cooking Time: 10 + 30mins

Total Time: 55mins

Instructions:

- In a medium mixing bowl, combine Worcestershire sauce, vinegar, soy sauce, chili powder, garlic, and hot pepper sauce.
- Turn the chicken in the sauce to coat. Marinate for 30 minutes at room temperature, or cover and refrigerate for several hours.
- In a large skillet, heat the oil over high heat.
- Cook and stir for 5 minutes in heated oil with chicken strips.
- Make sure to sauté the green pepper and onion for three minutes. Remove from the fire and season with lemon juice.

- Calories: 210 kcal
- Carbohydrate: 6g
- Fats: 8g
- Protein: 28g

33. Kale & Tuna Salad

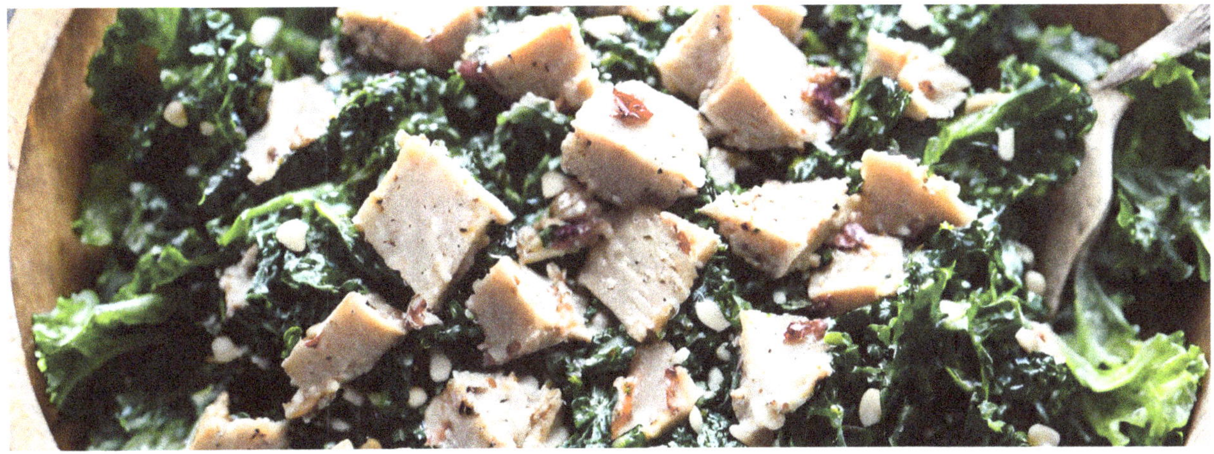

Ingredients:

- 2 tuna cans (5 oz. each)
- 1 bundle (or 1 bag) kale
- 2 oz. cherry tomatoes
- 1 raw lemon
- 1 tablespoon extra virgin olive oil
- 1 tbsp balsamic vinegar
- kosher salt (as desired)
- freshly ground pepper (as desired)

Prep Time: 15 mins **Serves:** 5

Cooking Time: 10 + 30mins

Total Time: 55mins

Nutritional Value

- Calories: 278 kcal
- Carbohydrate: 16g
- Fats: 16g
- Protein: 28g

Instructions:

- Kale should be washed. Set aside to drain the water.
- Toss tomatoes in a bowl with balsamic vinegar, olive oil, and a touch of salt and pepper. Place aside.
- In a salad dish, carefully combine tuna and can liquid with a squeeze of 1/2 lemon and a pinch of pepper.
- To soften the kale, massage it for about 3 minutes.
- To the tuna, add the kale and half of the tomatoes. Toss gently until evenly coated with dressing.
- Mix in the remaining tomatoes.
- Serve with the remaining lemon wedge.

34. Steak With Roasted Veggies

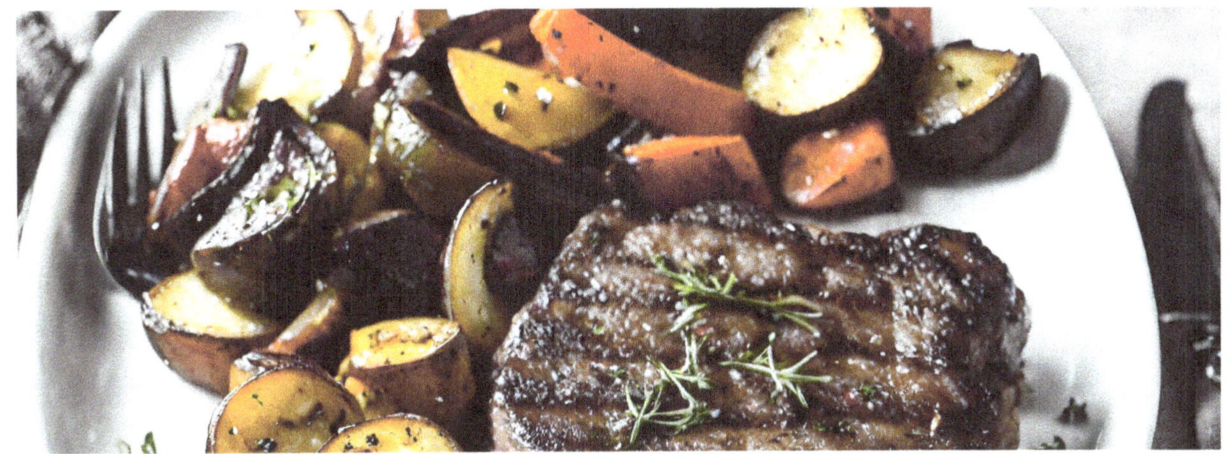

Ingredients:

Veggies

- 2 zucchini, cut in half circles
- 2 yellow squash, cut in half circles
- ½ pint grape or cherry tomatoes
- 1 red onion, thinly sliced
- 3 tablespoons olive or avocado oil
- ½ teaspoon garlic powder
- ½ teaspoon dried oregano
- ½ teaspoon salt

Steak

- 1 lb sirloin steak, finely divided into ½-inch thick chunks
- 2 tablespoons coconut aminos (or soy sauce)
- ½ teaspoon salt
- ½ teaspoon pepper
- ¼ tablespoon crushed red pepper flakes
- ¼ teaspoon garlic powder

Instructions:

- Preheat the oven to 425 degrees Fahrenheit. Line a baking sheet 12" x 17" with parchment paper.
- Combine steak, coconut aminos, salt, pepper, crushed red pepper flakes, and garlic powder in a mixing bowl. Place aside. (While you can marinate for up to 12 hours, this recipe does not require it. Allow it to marinate in the marinade ingredients while your vegetables cook.
- On a baking sheet, arrange the zucchini, squash, red onion, and tomatoes. They don't have to be kept apart. Dress with olive oil. Garlic powder, dried oregano, and salt to taste. Make sure everything

Prep Time: 5 mins   **Serves:** 4

Cooking Time: 25 mins

Total Time: 30 mins

Nutritional Value

- Calories: 311 kcal
- Carbohydrate: 11g
- Fats: 14g
- Protein: 28g

- is well-seasoned. After stirring, spread in a single layer.
- Bake for 20 minutes, or until the vegetables are softened and nearly done.
- Place the marinated steak on a baking sheet with the vegetables. Bake for 5 to 8 minutes, or until the steak is done to your liking.

35. Citrus Baked Fish

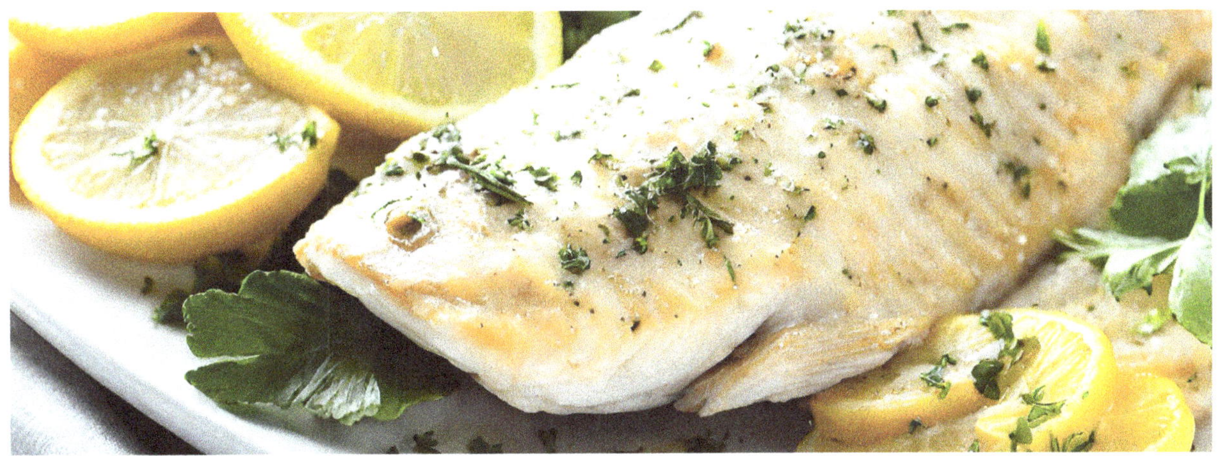

Ingredients:

- sprayed frying oil
- 4 salmon filets (3 ounces)
- ¼ cup fresh lemon juice
- ¼ cup of orange juice
- ¼ cup lemon juice
- 2 tbsp. melted butter
- 1 tsp. dried parsley
- ½ teaspoon paprika powder
- ¼ teaspoon salt
- ¼ teaspoon black pepper

Prep Time: 15 mins   **Serves:** 4

Cooking Time: 10 mins

Total Time: 25 mins

Nutritional Value

- Calories: 157 kcal
- Carbohydrate: 5g
- Fats: 7g
- Protein: 19g

Instructions:

- Preheat the oven to 350 degrees Fahrenheit (175 degrees Celsius). Lightly coat a baking dish with cooking spray.
- Fill the baking dish halfway with salmon filets.
- Mix together the lemon juice, orange juice, lime juice, butter, parsley, paprika, salt, and pepper until well combined. Pour over the fish in the baking dish.
- Bake fish in a preheated oven for 10 to 15 minutes, or until readily flaked with a fork. A thermometer inserted into the center should read 145 degrees Fahrenheit (63 degrees Celsius).

36. Spicy Salmon

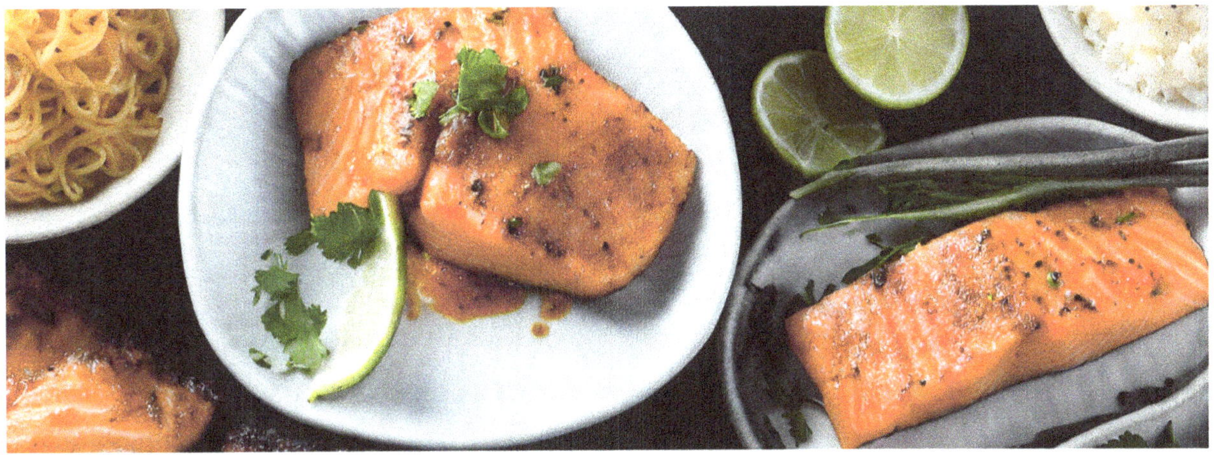

Ingredients:

- If feasible, get a 1¾-pound side of wild-caught salmon (skin on or off; if I'm not in a rush, I ask the seafood counter to remove the skin, but both work nicely).
- 1 tablespoon brown sugar optional; eliminate if following a Paleo or Whole30 diet.
- 1½ tsp chipotle chile powder
- 1 tablespoon lime juice
- 1 medium lime zest
- 1 tablespoon extra-virgin olive oil or melted unsalted butter
- 1½ tablespoons kosher salt
- 3 tbsp fresh cilantro, chopped

Prep Time: 5 mins   **Serves:** 4
Cooking Time: 15 mins
Total Time: 20 mins

Instructions:

- Remove the salmon from the refrigerator and set it aside for 10 minutes to come to room temperature while you prepare the other ingredients. Preheat the oven to 375°F. Line a large baking dish or rimmed baking sheet with aluminum foil large enough to wrap all the way around and seal the fish. Coat the foil lightly with nonstick spray. Pat the salmon dry with paper towels. Place the salmon in the center of the plate.
- Combine the brown sugar, chipotle chili powder, lime zest, and salt in a small mixing basin. Brush the fish with the lime juice and olive oil (or melted butter).

- Sprinkle the chipotle seasoning mixture over the salmon, pressing it in to coat evenly.
- Fold the aluminum foil sides up and over the top of the salmon until completely encased. If your piece of foil is too small, add another piece on top and fold the sides under to form a sealed packet. Allow some space inside the foil for air to flow.
- Bake the salmon for 12 to 18 minutes, or until the thickest part is almost entirely cooked through. Cooking time will vary according to the thickness of the fish. Check early to ensure your salmon does not overcook if your side is thinner (about 1 inch thick). If your item is particularly thick (1 1/2 inch or more), it may require more time.
- Remove the salmon from the oven and carefully remove the foil, exposing the top of the fish (be careful of hot steam). Change the oven setting to broil, then return the salmon to the oven for 3 minutes, or until the top is slightly brown and the fish is cooked through. Keep an eye on the salmon while it boils to ensure it does not overcook. Take the fish out of the oven. If it still seems underdone, wrap the foil around the top and set it aside for a few minutes. Do not let it sit for too long—salmon may easily go from not done to overcooked. It's done when it flakes easily with a fork. You can also use an instant-read thermometer to check the temperature of the fish. It's done when the temperature reaches 145 degrees F.
- Cut the salmon into chunks to serve. As desired, garnish with fresh cilantro or an extra squeeze of lime juice.

Nutritional Value

- Calories: 329 kcal
- Carbohydrate: 4g
- Fats: 16g
- Protein: 40g

37. Cauliflower Risotto

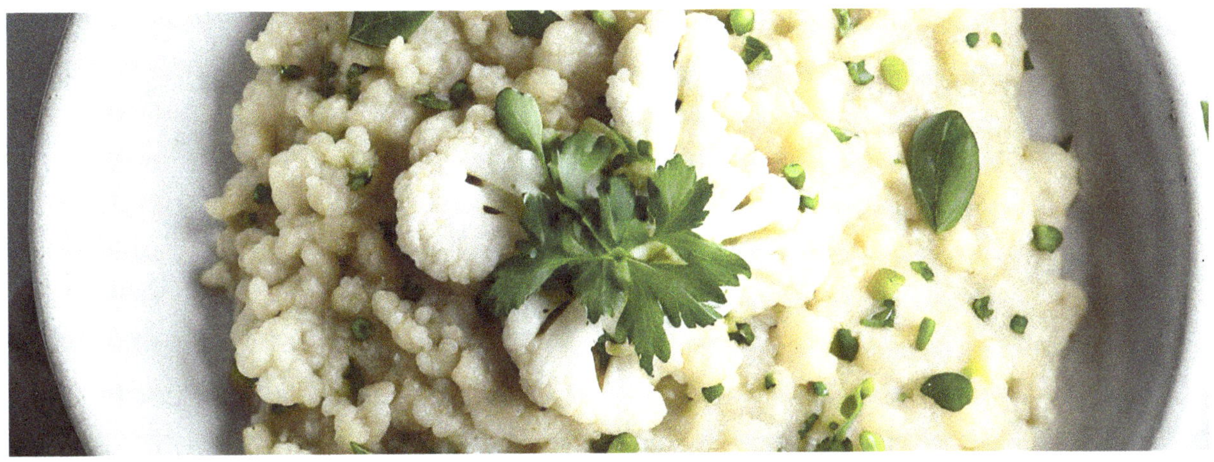

Ingredients:

- 1 cup white onions, diced (typically about one medium onion)
- 2 cups baby Portobello mushrooms, sliced
- 1 cauliflower head
- 2 Tbsp olive oil
- 2 Tbsp butter
- 1 cup vegetable stock
- 8 ounce Mascarpone cheese
- ½ cup grated Parmigiano-Reggiano
- Salt and pepper to taste

Prep Time: 15 mins   **Serves:** 6
Cooking Time: 15 mins
Total Time: 30 mins

Instructions:

- Prep your cauliflower. Remove green leaves and cut the cauliflower in half. Cut or break the florets from the stem and discard the stem.
- Add a handful of florets to a food processor or high speed blender until the container is about half way full. Pulse until the florets resemble a grain, then pour into a bowl.
- Repeat this process with the remaining cauliflower florets, only pulsing a handful at a time so that they're evenly chopped.
- Heat olive oil and butter in a large saute pan. Once oil is heated and butter is melted, add the onions

- Calories: 325 kcal
- Carbohydrate: 12g
- Fats: 29g
- Protein: 8g

- and mushrooms and cook until browned. Gently drain any excess water from the pan into the sink or a bowl.
- Once the excess water is drained, add the cauliflower and vegetable stock. Bring heat to a boil, then reduce to medium to simmer. Stir continuously and cook on medium heat until cauliflower is tender and the stock is reduced.
- Next, spoon the mascarpone cheese over the cauliflower until it's melted, creating a cheesy sauce.
- Sprinkle with Parmigiano-Reggiano, then add a pinch of salt and pepper to taste.
- Garnish with chopped parsley and serve with your favorite wine.

38. Mediterranean Wings

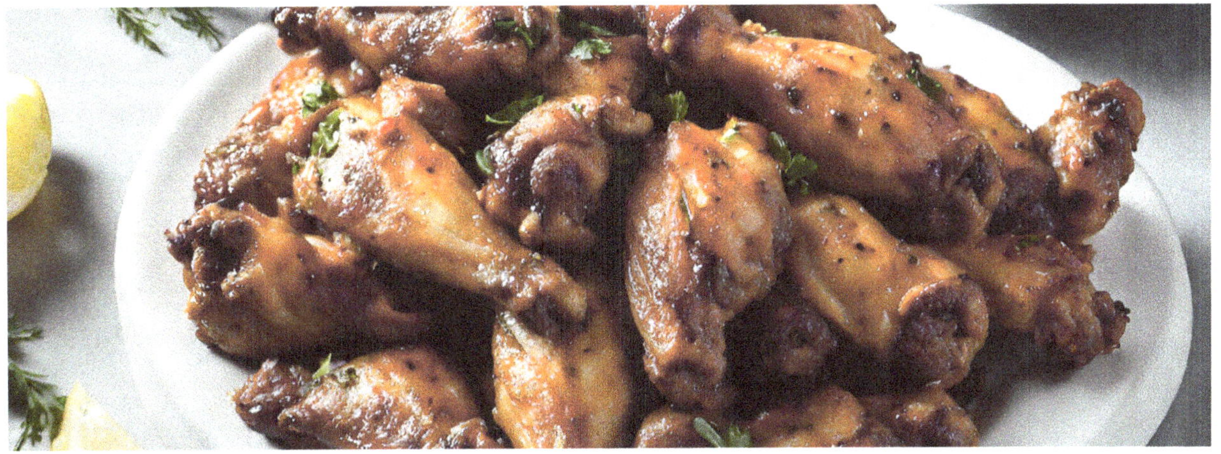

Ingredients:

- 2 pound chicken wings, split at joints, tips removed
- 2 tbsp of olive oil
- 2 teaspoons oregano, dried
- 1 teaspoon thyme dried
- 1 smoked paprika teaspoon
- 1 teaspoon cumin powder
- 1 tsp. garlic powder
- Season with salt and pepper to taste.
- 1 sliced lemon
- Garnish with fresh parsley

Prep Time: 15 mins   **Serves:** 4

Cooking Time: 45 mins

Total Time: 60 mins

Instructions:

- Preheat the oven to 400 degrees Fahrenheit (200 degrees Celsius). Line a baking sheet using a parchment paper
- Toss chicken wings with olive oil, dried oregano, dried thyme, smoked paprika, ground cumin, garlic powder, salt, and pepper in a large mixing bowl. Make certain that the wings are evenly coated.
- Arrange the seasoned chicken wings in a single layer on the prepared baking sheet.
- Distribute the lemon slices evenly on top of the wings.
- Bake for approximately 40 minutes, or until the wings are golden brown and crispy. For

Nutritional Value

- Calories: 350 kcal
- Carbohydrate: 2g
- Fats: 27g
- Protein: 25g

- even browning, flip the wings halfway through the cooking time.
- Remove from the oven and set aside for a few minutes to cool.
- Garnish the Mediterranean Chicken Wings with fresh parsley and serve with Greek yogurt or tzatziki for dipping.

39. Salmon Salad Wraps

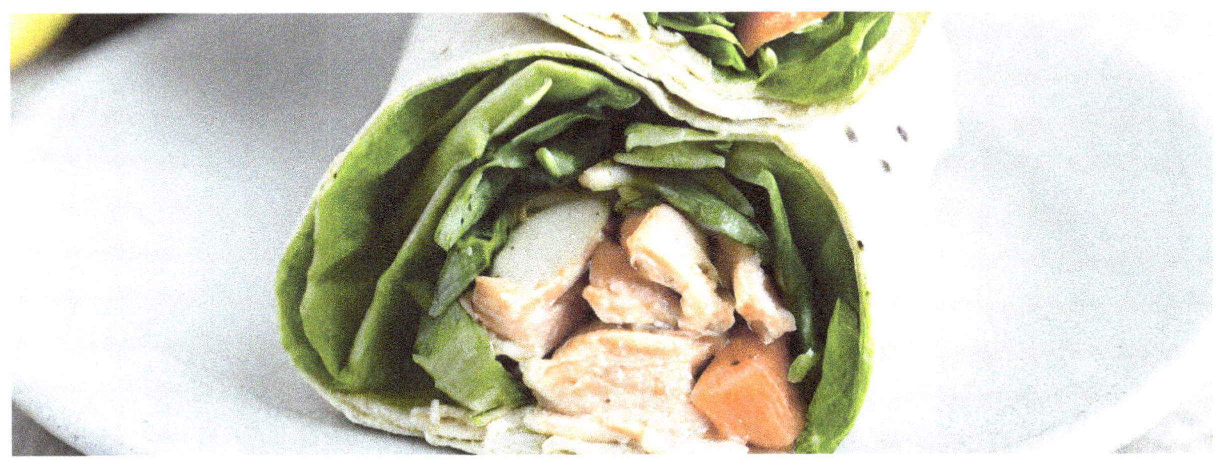

Ingredients:

- 1 (14.75-oz.) can flaked red sockeye salmon
- 1 cup cucumber, diced
- ¼ cup green onions, chopped
- ¼ cup fresh dill, chopped
- 1 medium chopped red bell pepper
- 1 can whole kernel sweet corn (11 oz.)
- ½ cup store-bought ranch salad dressing
- 5 huge leaf lettuce leaves
- 5 burrito or wrap-size wheat tortillas (10 to 12 inches)

Prep Time: 20 mins **Serves:** 4
Cooking Time: 0 mins
Total Time: 20 mins

Instructions:

- In a medium mixing bowl, combine all ingredients except the lettuce and tortillas.
- To soften the tortillas, heat them as instructed on the package.
- Each tortilla should have a lettuce leaf down the center. Distribute 1 cup of the salmon mixture equally over the lettuce.
- Fold the bottom 14 of each tortilla up; fold the sides toward the center.

Nutritional Value

- Calories: 510 kcal
- Carbohydrate: 6g
- Fats: 25g
- Protein: 53g

40. Cheesy Salmon

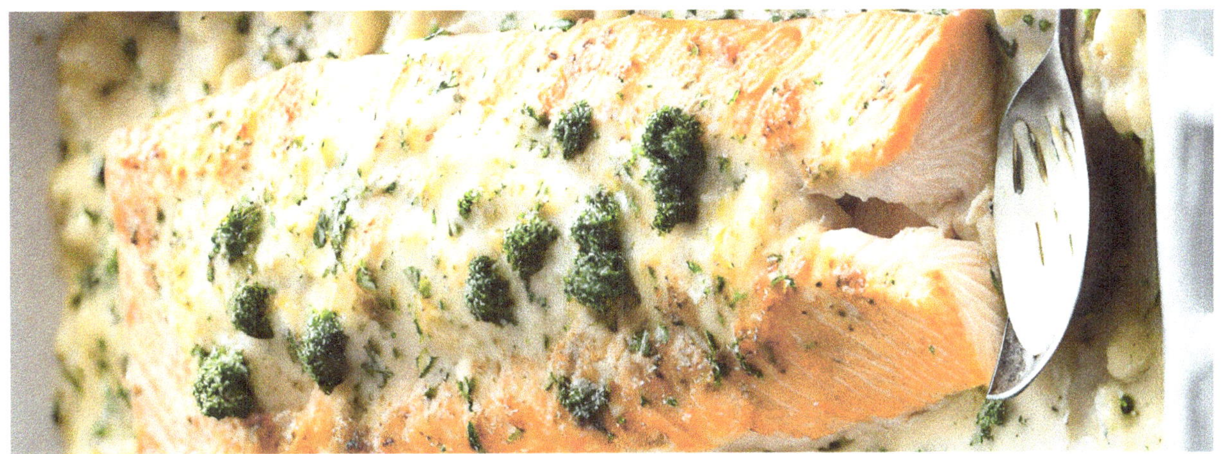

Ingredients:

- Four skinless, roughly 6-ounce salmon filets.
- 1 cup low-fat mozzarella cheese, shredded
- ¼ cup Parmesan cheese, grated
- 2 tbsp of olive oil
- 2 tbsp fresh parsley, chopped
- 1 tsp. garlic powder
- 1 tsp. onion powder
- Season with salt and pepper to taste.
- Optional lemon wedges for serving

Prep Time: 15 mins   **Serves:** 4

Cooking Time: 25 mins

Total Time: 40 mins

Instructions:

- Set the oven's temperature to 375° F. (190 degrees Celsius). Line a baking dish with parchment paper.
- Place the salmon filets in the baking dish that has been prepared. Each filet should be seasoned with salt, pepper, garlic powder, and onion powder.
- In a small mixing dish, combine the shredded mozzarella and grated Parmesan cheeses.
- Drizzle olive oil over the salmon filets to cover completely.
- Evenly distribute the cheese mixture over the salmon filets.
- Bake for 15-20 minutes, or until the salmon is cooked through and

- the cheese is golden brown and bubbling, in a preheated oven.
- Remove the roasted salmon from the oven and top with chopped fresh parsley.
- If desired, serve the salmon filets with lemon wedges on the side.

41. Steamed Garlic Chicken Breasts

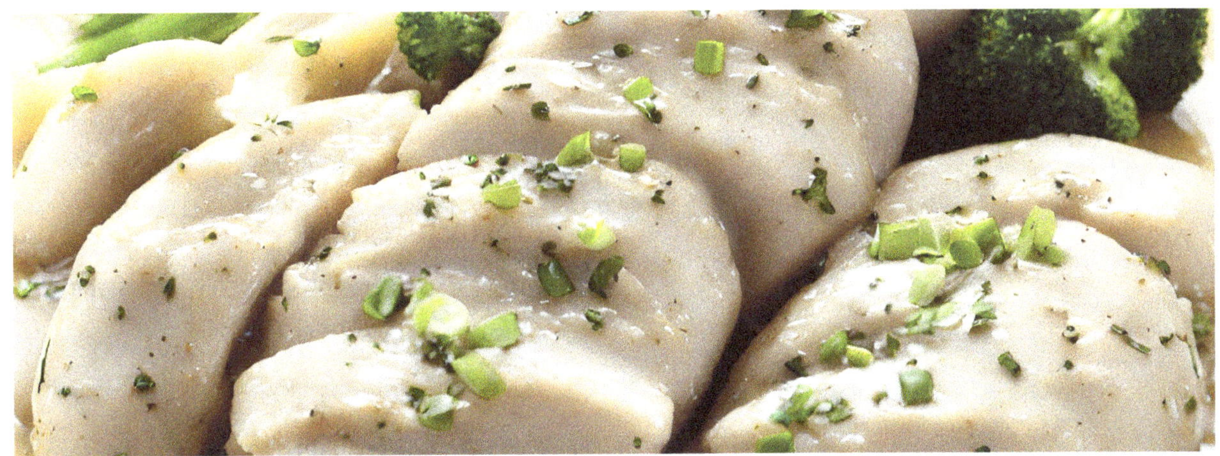

Ingredients:

- 4 boneless, skinless chicken breasts (about 1.5 pounds)
- 6 minced garlic cloves
- 2 tbsp. low-sodium soy sauce
- 1 tbsp sesame seed oil
- 1 tablespoon vinegar (rice)
- 1 teaspoon fresh ginger, grated
- 1 tablespoon honey
- ½ teaspoon ground black pepper
- For garnish, use green onions (scallions).
- Optional garnish: sesame seeds

Prep Time: 15 mins   **Serves:** 4
Cooking Time: 20 mins
Total Time: 35 mins

Instructions:

- Prepare the chicken breasts by patting them dry with paper towels.
- To make the marinade, combine minced garlic, soy sauce, sesame oil, rice vinegar, grated ginger, honey, and black pepper in a small bowl.
- Marinating the Chicken: In a shallow dish, coat the chicken breasts equally with the marinade. Allow at least 15 minutes for it to marinade.
- Prepare a steamer for steaming. If you don't have a steamer, a large pot with a steamer basket will suffice.
- Place the marinated chicken

Nutritional Value

- Calories: 200 kcal
- Carbohydrate: 7g
- Fats: 7g
- Protein: 30g

- breasts on the rack of a steamer.
- The chicken should be cooked thoroughly after 20 minutes of steaming. Check that the interior temperature is 165°F (74°C).
- Garnish the steamed garlic chicken breasts with chopped green onions and sesame seeds, if desired.
- Serve the chicken breasts with steamed veggies or brown rice on the side.

42. Lemon Garlic Shrimp And Asparagus

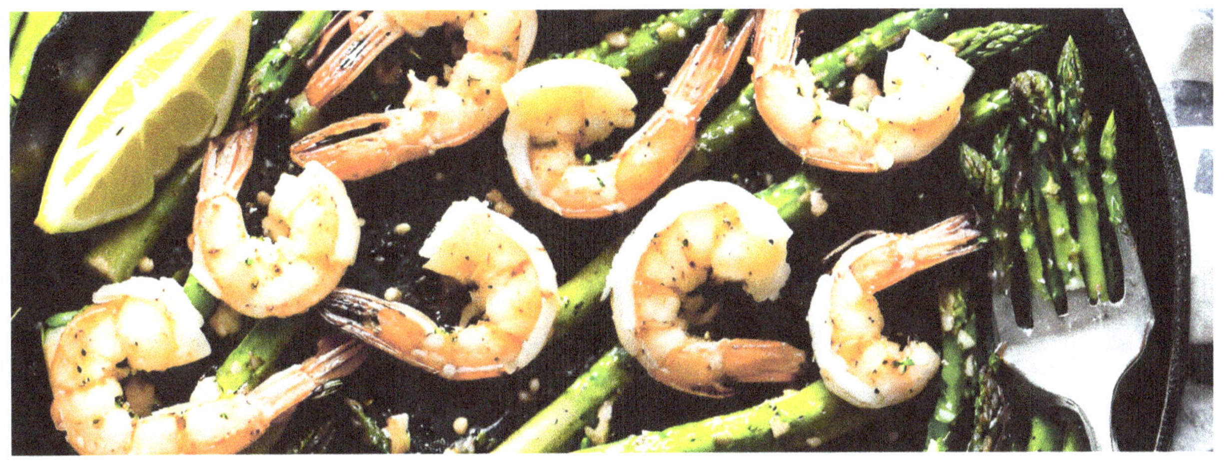

Ingredients:

- cooking spray
- 1 pound fresh asparagus, trimmed
- 2 tablespoons olive oil, divided
- 4 cloves garlic, minced salt, divided
- 1 pinch powdered black pepper, divided
- 1½ pounds uncooked medium shrimp, skinned and deveined
- 1 teaspoon paprika
- 3 tbsp. butter
- 3 tbsp. lemon juice

Prep Time: 10 mins   **Serves:** 4
Cooking Time: 12 mins
Total Time: 22 mins

Instructions:

- Preheat the oven to 400°F (200°C). Line a rimmed 9x12-inch baking pan with parchment paper and coat with cooking spray.
- Place the asparagus on the prepared baking sheet and drizzle with 1 tablespoon olive oil. Toss with garlic, 1 teaspoon salt, and ½ teaspoon pepper until well covered. Arrange the asparagus in a single layer.
- 6 minutes in a preheated oven until slightly tender.
- Remove from the oven and arrange the shrimp on one side of the pan. Toss with the remaining 1 tablespoon olive oil, 1 teaspoon salt, 1/2 teaspoon pepper, and

Nutritional Value

- Calories: 300 kcal
- Carbohydrate: 7g
- Fats: 17g
- Protein: 31g

- smoked paprika until completely coated. Arrange the shrimp in a single layer next to the asparagus. Cubed butter should be drizzled over the asparagus and shrimp.
- 6 minutes in a preheated oven until the shrimp are opaque.
- Remove the skillet from the oven and sprinkle with lemon juice.

43. Vegan Stuffed Potatoes With Quinoa

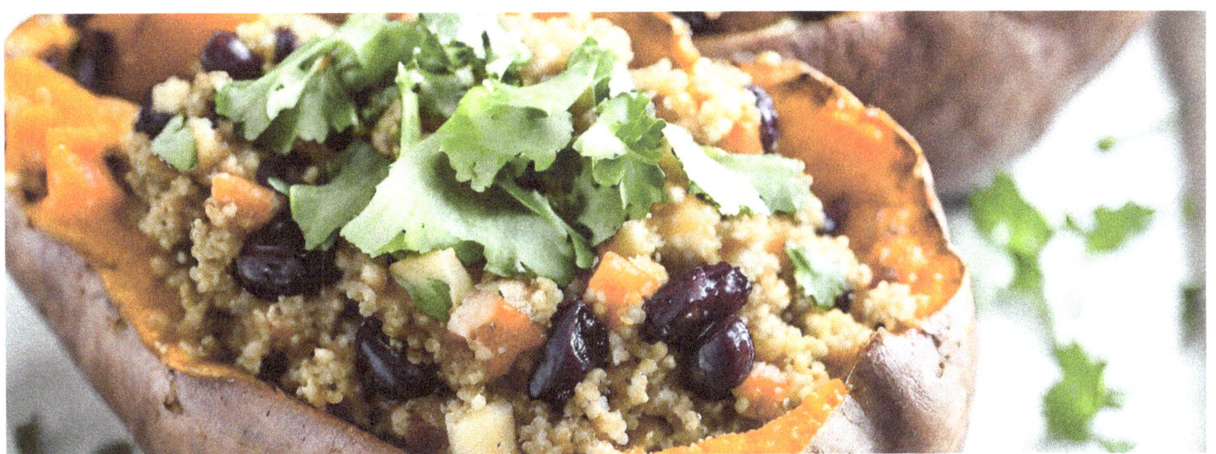

Ingredients:

- 2 medium sized sweet potatoes
- 1 tablespoon extra virgin olive oil
- 2 cups of spinach
- ½ cup chickpeas, canned
- ¼ cup chopped sun-dried tomatoes
- 2 tablespoons chopped kalamata olives
- 1 cup quinoa, cooked
- ½ tsp dried thyme
- ½ tsp dried dill
- ½ tsp garlic powder

To Garnish

- season with salt and pepper to taste.
- 1 teaspoon tahini
- 1 tsp. lemon juice
- 1 tsp salt and pepper
- 1 – 2 tbsp water to thin chives
- flakes of red pepper

Instructions:

- Preheat the oven to 400 degrees Fahrenheit. Place the sweet potatoes in a baking tray and poke them with a fork. Bake until tender and the knife easily slides into the flesh, 35-45 minutes depending on size.
- Meanwhile, heat the oil in a saute pan over medium heat for the quinoa mixture. Sauté the remaining ingredients (spinach, salt, and pepper) until heated. Warm until the sweet potatoes are tender.
- Remove the sweet potatoes from the oven and set aside for a few minutes to cool. Transfer to a platter, split open with a sharp

Prep Time: 5 mins   **Serves:** 2

Cooking Time: 45 mins

Total Time: 50 mins

Nutritional Value

- Calories: 423 kcal
- Carbohydrate: 63g
- Fats: 15g
- Protein: 13g

- knife, and ladle the quinoa into the center.
- Pour the tahini, lemon, salt, pepper, and water mixture over the sweet potatoes. Garnish with chives and red pepper flakes if desired. Serve right away and enjoy!

44. Beef & Broccoli Stir-fry with Jasmine Rice

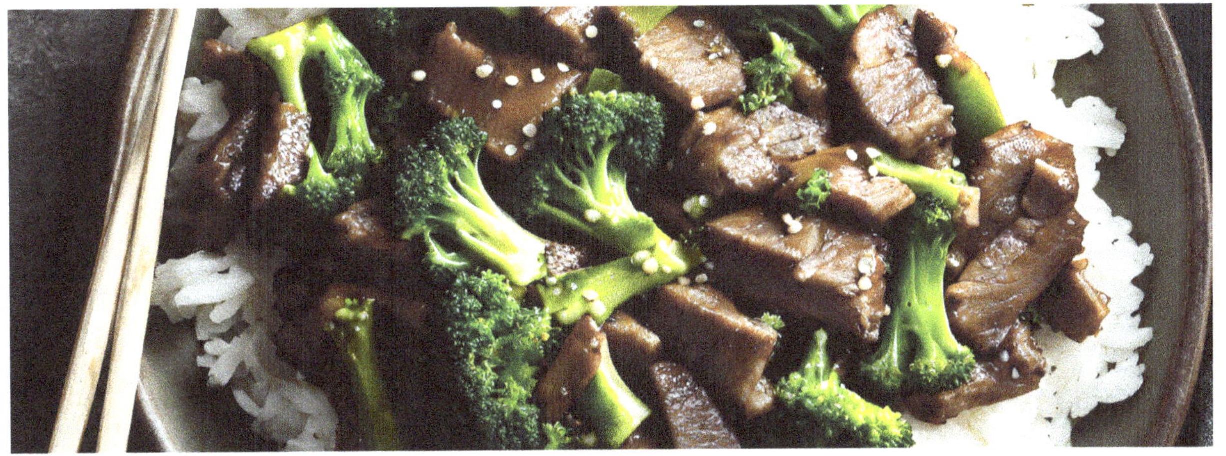

Ingredients:

- 1 (14.75-oz.) can flaked red sockeye salmon
- 1 cup cucumber, diced
- ¼ cup green onions, chopped
- ¼ cup fresh dill, chopped
- 1 medium chopped red bell pepper
- 1 can whole kernel sweet corn (11 oz.)
- ½ cup store-bought ranch salad dressing
- 5 huge leaf lettuce leaves
- 5 burrito or wrap-size wheat tortillas (10 to 12 inches)

Prep Time: 10 mins   **Serves:** 4
Cooking Time: 20 mins
Total Time: 30 mins

Instructions:

- Spray a large skillet with nonstick cooking spray and brown the steak.
- Sauté for 1 minute with the garlic, green onion, broccoli, and soy sauce.
- Cook rice according per package directions.
- Serve the beef and broccoli over rice or as a single dish.

Nutritional Value

- Calories: 850 kcal
- Carbohydrate: 73g
- Fats: 50g
- Protein: 36g

45. Grilled Chicken Caesar Salad

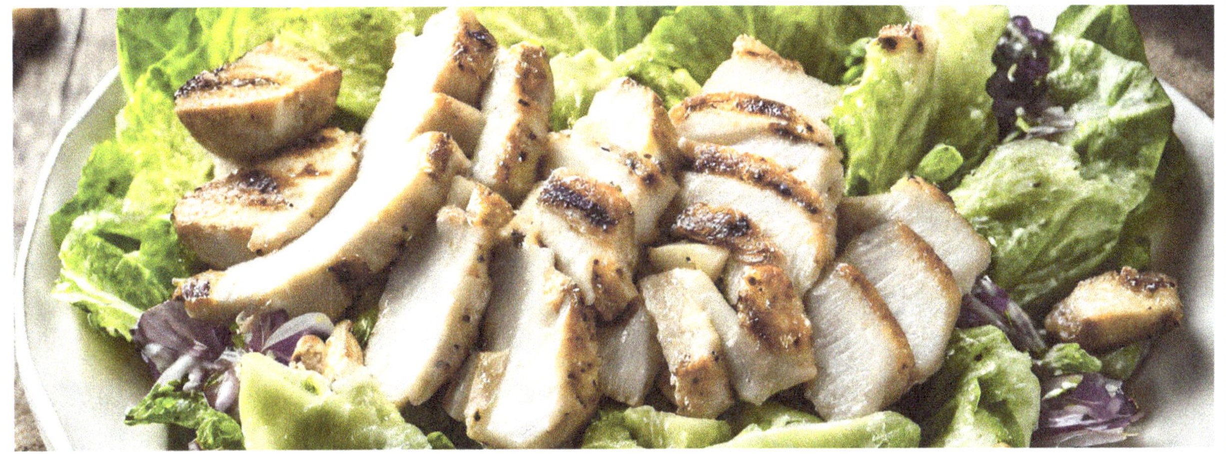

Ingredients:

- 1 - 1¼ lb of boneless chicken breast
- 2 tablespoons lemon juice or red wine vinegar
- 2 teaspoon olive oil
- ½ tsp garlic powder
- ½ tsp dried thyme
- ½ tsp dried oregano
- ¼ teaspoon pepper
- ¼ teaspoon salt

Salad
- Croutons made from sourdough
- Caesar Dressing
- 1 romaine lettuce head, cut into bite-sized pieces
- Shaved fresh parmesan

Instructions:

- In a small mixing bowl, add vinegar, oil, garlic powder, thyme, oregano, salt, and pepper.
- Fill a shallow dish or a 1-gallon sealable plastic bag halfway with chicken. Refrigerate for at least 1 hour or up to 12 hours after adding the marinade.
- Bake the sourdough croutons while the chicken marinates.
- While the croutons are baking, make the dressing by combining all of the ingredients and blending until thick and creamy.
- Remove the chicken from the marinade, shaking off any excess, and discard any remaining marinade. Preheat your grill or

Prep Time: 20 mins   **Serves:** 2

Cooking Time: 25 mins

Total Time: 45 mins

Nutritional Value

- Calories: 575 kcal
- Carbohydrate: 19g
- Fats: 30g
- Protein: 57g

- grill pan. Once the grill is hot, cook the chicken for about 5 minutes per side, or until cooked through and no longer pink. The chicken's internal temperature should be 165°F.
- Salad is ready when you add a bed of romaine lettuce to two bowls. Sliced chicken breast, sourdough croutons, and shaved parmesan are optional. Drizzle with Caesar dressing and serve immediately.

Dessert Ideas for a Healthy Diet

46. Mixed Berry and Chia Seed Pudding

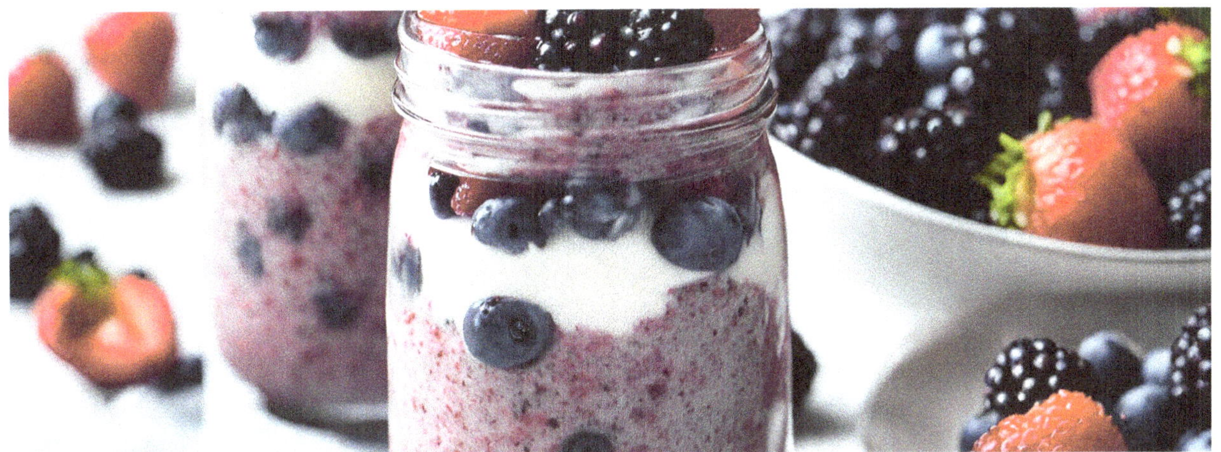

Ingredients:

- 2 cups divided organic mixed berries
- ¾ cup full fat coconut milk (add an additional ¼ cup coconut milk for a creamier texture)
- ½ cup of chia seeds
- ½ teaspoon genuine vanilla extract
- ½ teaspoon cinnamon powder
- ½ tsp of sea salt
- ½ cup unsweetened shredded coconut
- 2 tbsp of hemp seeds
- ¼ cup chopped toasted pumpkin seeds or other nut

Instructions:

- Blend 1 cup of the berries and the coconut milk in a stand up or hand blender until smooth.
- Combine the chia seeds, vanilla essence, cinnamon, and salt in a medium mixing dish. Stir in the berry coconut mixture until completely blended. Cover tightly and place in the refrigerator for at least 12 hours.
- When ready to serve, divide the mixture among four bowls and top with the coconut, hemp seeds, seeds or almonds, and the remaining 1 cup of berries.

Prep Time: 10 mins   **Serves:** 4

Resting Time: 12 hrs

Total Time: 12 hrs 10 mins

Nutritional Value

- Calories: 391kcal
- Carbohydrate: 24g
- Fats: 31g
- Protein: 10g

47. Almond and Date Energy Balls

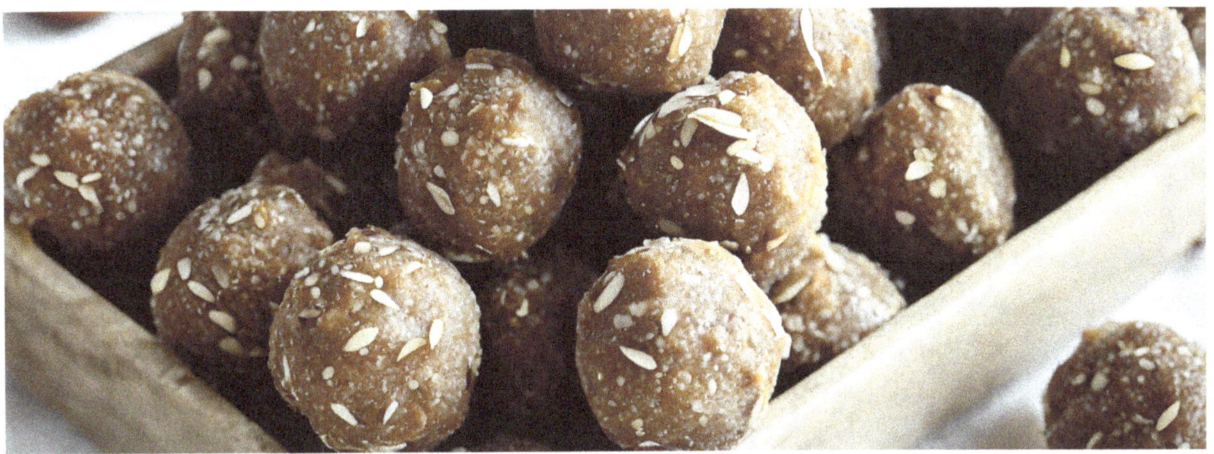

Ingredients:

- 10 Medjool Dates (pitted and diced)
- 1 cup Almonds, roasted
- ½ cup flaked unsweetened coconut
- ¼ cup Almond Butter
- 1 tablespoon Rodelle Cinnamon Ceylon
- a dash of sea salt
- (for rolling) ¾ cup unsweetened shredded coconut

Prep Time: 10 mins
Cooking Time: 0 mins
Total Time: 10 mins

Serves: 12 balls

Instructions:

- In a food processor, finely grind dates, almonds, 12 cup coconut, almond butter, cinnamon, and salt.
- Make walnut-sized balls out of the mixture.
- Take each ball and roll it with shredded coconut. Roll again to create balls. Place on a baking sheet with a rim and lined with wax paper.
- Refrigerate for 30 minutes before placing in an airtight container. Stop the fridge or freezer. (If freezing, take as many as you need from the freezer, thaw, and then store in the refrigerator for snacking.)

- Calories: 180 kcal
- Carbohydrate: 14g
- Fats: 10g
- Protein: 5g

48. Dark Chocolate and Avocado Moussece

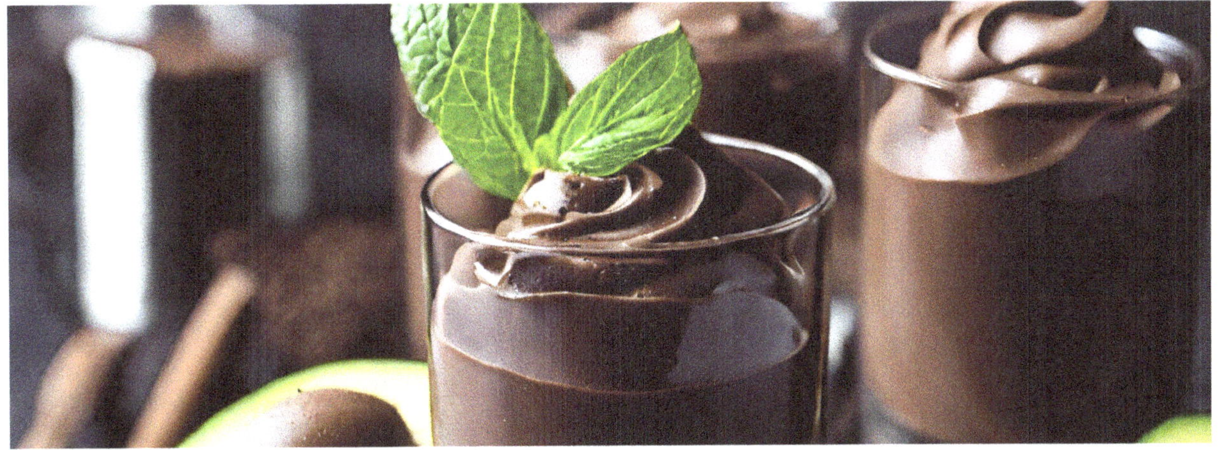

Ingredients:

- 2 avocados that are very ripe
- ¼ cup unsweetened cocoa powder, melted
- 4 ounces 70% cacao baking chocolate
- ⅓ cup of almond milk
- ⅓ cup pure maple syrup
- ½ tsp vanilla extract
- ¼ teaspoon ground cinnamon
- Sea salt
- Toppings are optional and may include chocolate whipped cream or coconut whipped cream, roughly chopped dark chocolate, berries, almonds, and so on.

Prep Time: 10 mins   **Serves:** 4
Cooking Time: 0 mins
Total Time: 10 mins

Instructions:

- Combine the avocados, melted chocolate, cocoa powder, maple syrup, almond milk, vanilla, cinnamon, and a bit of salt in a food processor. Puree till smooth. Chill the mousse in 4 tiny ramekins for at least 1 hour.
- Serve the mousse topped with whipped cream and/or your preferred garnishes.

Notes

- If making this vegan, use dairy-free chocolate.
- I made chocolate whipped cream by using this recipe for homemade whipped cream with 1 tablespoon

- Calories: 295 kcal
- Carbohydrate: 32g
- Fats: 19g
- Protein: 4g

49. Mango Coconut Chia Pudding

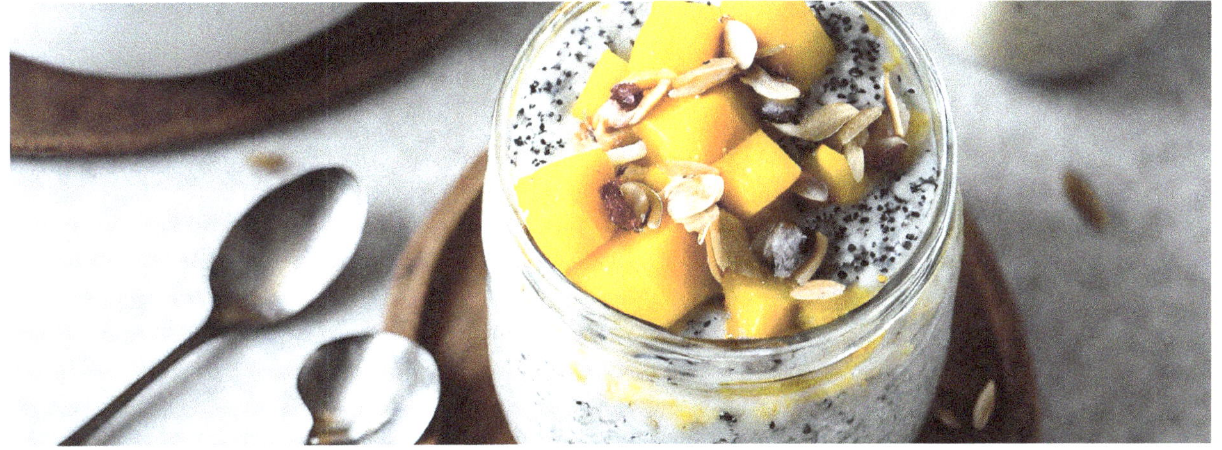

Ingredients:

- ½ cup unsweetened coconut milk
- ½ cup almond milk, unsweetened
- ¾ cup sliced fresh ripe champagne mango
- 4 tablespoons chia seeds
- 1 tablespoon shredded sweetened coconut
- 4-6 drops Nu-Naturals liquid stevia or monk fruit, to taste sugar/honey

Instructions:

- In a large mixing bowl, combine all of the ingredients. Allow to settle for 30 minutes before mixing again. Refrigerate for at least 5-6 hours, or overnight, until the seeds expand and thicken.
- Serve in two separate bowls or glass dishes. Enjoy!

Prep Time: 5 mins   **Serves:** 2
Chill Time: 5 hrs
Total Time: 5 hrs 5 mins

Nutritional Value

- Calories: 227 kcal
- Carbohydrate: 22g
- Fats: 13g
- Protein: 7g

50. Peanut Butter Oatmeal Balls

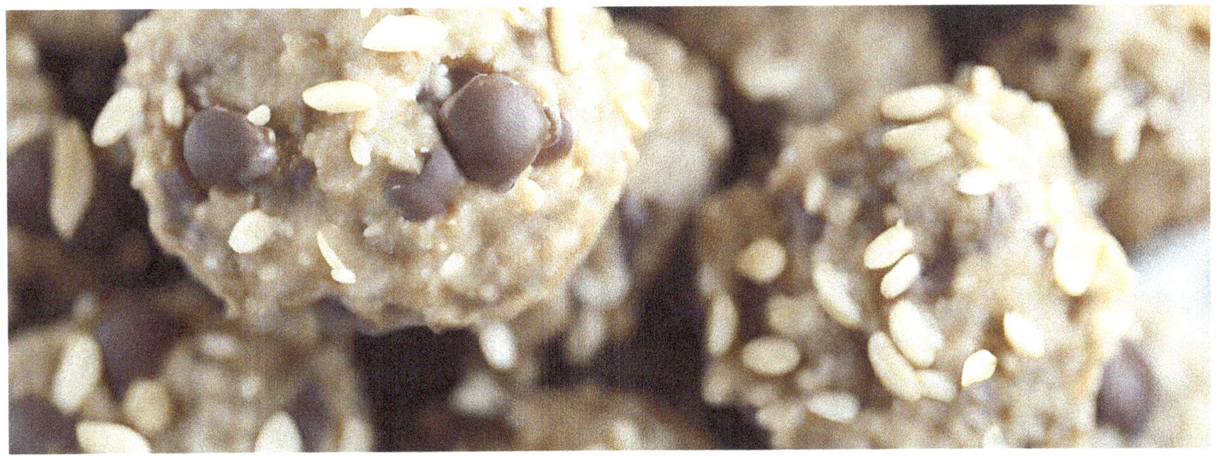

Ingredients:

- 1⅓ cup (120 g) gluten-free rolled oats
- 2 tbsp (20 g) the seeds of chia
- ⅓ cup (80 g) creamy peanut butter or your favorite nut/seed butter
- ¼ cup (80 g) maple syrup or your preferred liquid sweetener
- 3 Tbsp (30 g) Optional dairy-free chocolate chips

Prep Time: 10 mins

Chill Time: 15 mins

Total Time: 25 mins

Serves: 11 balls

Instructions:

- To begin, soften the peanut butter in a double boiler or microwave. Allow it to cool.
- You can omit this step if the peanut butter is already fluid (as in natural peanut butter).
- Then, in a medium mixing dish, add the oats and chia seeds. Stir in the runny peanut butter, sugar, and chocolate chips (if using) until thoroughly blended.
- Refrigerate the mixing dish for about 15 minutes to help the mixture firm up (essential for rolling the balls easily).
- Divide the mixture with a tiny ice cream scoop (or cookie scoop) and roll it with your hands (oil

Nutritional Value

- Calories: 113 kcal
- Carbohydrate: 12.5g
- Fats: 5g
- Protein: 3.4g

- your hands if necessary). There was enough dough to make 11 balls.
- You may eat the peanut butter oat energy balls right away or place them in the refrigerator to firm up a little more.

Conclusion

In the culminating pages of this comprehensive guide, we find ourselves at the intersection of knowledge and action, armed with insights to fortify the guardian of our internal health – the liver. As we reflect upon the journey through the intricacies of fatty liver disease and the transformative potential of mindful dietary choices, let us distill the essence of our exploration.

Understanding the Power of Nutrition:
Throughout these chapters, we delved into the intricacies of non-alcoholic fatty liver disease (NAFLD), recognizing it not as a singular diagnosis but a call to embark on a journey of self-care. We deciphered the language of nutrients, unveiling the impact of wholesome choices on liver health.

The Fatty Liver Diet Unveiled:
The Fatty Liver Diet, presented with careful consideration for seniors and beginners, emerged as a roadmap to rejuvenation. From vibrant fruits to lean proteins, from leafy greens to heart-healthy fats, each ingredient is a note in the symphony of nourishment designed to support liver function.

A Culinary Odyssey:
Within these pages, recipes unfolded as a culinary odyssey – not a restrictive regimen but an invitation to savor the rich tapestry of flavors that contribute to well-being. Whether it's the crisp freshness of a salad or the warmth of a spiced stew, each dish embodies the fusion of nutrition and gastronomic delight.

The Art of Lifestyle Transformation:
Beyond the plate, we explored the art of lifestyle transformation. Exercise, hydration, and mindful habits emerged as allies in the pursuit of holistic health. The canvas of our well-being extends beyond the kitchen, inviting us to embrace a lifestyle that nurtures both body and spirit.

A Gentle Reminder:
As we bid farewell to these pages, let this be a gentle reminder – health is an ongoing journey, and every choice contributes to the narrative of our

well-being. Small, consistent steps yield enduring results. Prioritize whole foods, savor the joy of movement, and cultivate a mindset of self-care.

Tips for Lifelong Liver Wellness

1. Balanced Nutrition: Continue embracing a balanced diet rich in fruits, vegetables, lean proteins, and whole grains.

2. Hydration: Maintain optimal hydration by consuming an adequate amount of water throughout the day.

3. Physical Activity: Engage in regular physical activity tailored to your abilities and preferences.

4. Mindful Choices: Be mindful of processed foods, excessive sugars, and unhealthy fats. Opt for whole, nutrient-dense options.

5. Regular Check-ups: Schedule regular health check-ups to monitor liver function and overall well-being.

In summary, this book stands as a beacon of empowerment, guiding you towards a future where liver wellness is not just a goal but a lived reality. May these insights linger as you embark on a lifelong journey of nourishing your liver and, by extension, nurturing the vitality that resides within.

I Need Your Help

Dear Readers,

I hope you've embarked on a flavorful journey through the pages of my book, "Fatty Liver Diet Cookbook For Seniors And Beginners." Crafting this culinary exploration has been a labor of love, and I'm eager to hear your thoughts!

Your honest reviews play a crucial role in shaping not just my journey as an author but also in guiding fellow readers on their paths to wellness. Whether you found a particular recipe inspiring or discovered a new perspective on healthy living, your insights matter.

Take a moment to share your thoughts on Amazon. Your reviews are a beacon for others, helping them navigate the vast landscape of health-focused literature. Embrace the power of your words to foster a community dedicated to nourishing not just the body but the soul.

And if you'd like to stay connected, don't forget to follow my Author Central page for updates on upcoming books with exclusive content, and a behind-the-scenes look into the world of culinary wellness. Your support means the world to me, and I'm excited to continue this journey together.

Thank you for being a part of this flavorful adventure. Here's to savoring the richness of life and health!

My Deepest Gratitude

Dearest Reader,

As we come to an end of this fulfilling trip, I would like to express my deep thanks to you. I've prepared a special bonus for you as a thank you (I always keep my promises).

To get your bonus:
1. Scan the QR code that's right here in the middle of this page to obtain your bonus.
2. You'll be directed to a unique download page where your exclusive bonus is waiting for you.

This book was inspired by your passion for living a better lifestyle, and I'm excited to provide you with these extra tools.

Again, I appreciate that you selected the "Fatty Liver Diet Cookbook For Seniors and Beginners." May you have many satisfying and life-changing meals on your path to wellness.

Warm regards,
Juanita Scott.

Cooking Conversion Chart

Measurements

CUPS	OUNCES	MILLILITER	TABLESPOON
8 cups	64 oz	1895 mil	128
6 cups	48 oz	1420 mil	96
5 cups	40 oz	1120 mil	80
4 cups	32 oz	960 mil	64
2 cup	16 oz	480 mil	32
1 cup	8 oz	240 mil	16
¾ cup	6 oz	177 mil	12
⅔ cup	5 oz	158 mil	11
½ cup	4 oz	118 mil	8
⅜ cup	3 oz	90 mil	6
⅓ cup	2.5 oz	79 mil	5.5
¼ cup	2 oz	59 mil	4
⅛ cup	1 oz	30 mil	3
1/16 cup	½ oz	15 mil	1

Temperature

FAHRENHEIT	CELCIUS
100 °F	37 °C
150 °F	65 °C
200 °F	93 °C
250 °F	121 °C
300 °F	150 °C
325 °F	160 °C
350 °F	180 °C
375 °F	190 °C
400 °F	200 °C
425 °F	220 °C
450 °F	230 °C
500 °F	260 °C
525 °F	274 °C
550 °F	288 °C

Weight

IMPERIAL	METRIC
½ oz	15 g
1 oz	29 g
2 oz	57 g
3 oz	85 g
4 oz	113 g
5 oz	141 g
6 oz	170 g
8 oz	227 g
10 oz	283 g
12 oz	340 g
13 oz	369 g
14 oz	397 g
15 oz	425 g
1 lb	453 g

Bonus
MEAL PLAN

MONDAY

Breakfast	Chia Seeds Pudding
Lunch	Avocado & Lentil Power Bowl
Dinner	Pan Seared Salmon
Snack	Sliced Cucumber with Hummus

TUESDAY

Breakfast	Fruit Salad
Lunch	Broccoli and Cauliflower Stir Fry
Dinner	Pollo Fajitas
Snack	Greek Yogurt with a Handful of Nuts

WEDNESDAY

Breakfast	Guacamole Toast
Lunch	Vegetable Frittata
Dinner	Kale & Tuna Salad
Snack	Apple Slices with Almond Butter

THURSDAY

Breakfast	Homemade Oatmeal
Lunch	Chilled Tomato Gazpacho Soup
Dinner	Steak With Roasted Veggies
Snack	Carrot Sticks with Tzatziki

FRIDAY

Breakfast	Greek Yogurt and Berries
Lunch	Sweet Potato Vegan Buddha Bowl
Dinner	Citrus Baked Fish
Snack	Sliced Bell Peppers with Guacamole

SATURDAY

Breakfast	Mediterranean Quinoa Salad
Lunch	Salmon With Green Bean Almondine
Dinner	Spicy Salmon
Snack	Trail Mix with Nuts and Seeds

SUNDAY

Breakfast	Fresh Vegetable Salad
Lunch	Grilled Lemon Herb Chicken Salad
Dinner	Cauliflower Risotto
Snack	-

WATER INTAKE

MONDAY	
TUESDAY	
WEDNESDAY	
THURSDAY	
FRIDAY	
SATURDAY	
SUNDAY	

Bonus
MEAL PLAN

Week :

Date :

MONDAY

Breakfast	Skinny Omelet
Lunch	Banana Nut Muffins
Dinner	Mediterranean Wings
Snack	-

TUESDAY

Breakfast	Healthy Egg Muffins
Lunch	Spinach and Turkey Stuffed Peppers
Dinner	Salmon Salad Wraps
Snack	-

WEDNESDAY

Breakfast	Ricotta Avocado Toast
Lunch	Veggie-Packed Shrimp Spring Rolls
Dinner	Cheesy Salmon
Snack	-

THURSDAY

Breakfast	Tofu Scramble
Lunch	Eggplant Parmesan Stacks
Dinner	Steamed Garlic Chicken Breasts
Snack	-

FRIDAY

Breakfast	Vegan Waffles
Lunch	Balsamic Glazed Fish
Dinner	Lemon Garlic Shrimp & Asparagus
Snack	-

SATURDAY

Breakfast	Almond Butter and Banana Toast
Lunch	Greek Quesadillas
Dinner	Vegan Stuffed Sweet Potatoes with Quinoa
Snack	-

SUNDAY

Breakfast	Gluten-free Banana Pancakes
Lunch	Lean Turkey Paprikash
Dinner	Beef & Broccoli Stir-fry with Jasmine Rice
Snack	-

WATER INTAKE

MONDAY	
TUESDAY	
WEDNESDAY	
THURSDAY	
FRIDAY	
SATURDAY	
SUNDAY